apple Clary Mexican Roselea
o Spires Painted Autumn Rosy
Silver Jame Little a Bi
og Showy White Bee Commor
Wooly Cleveland Gentian Ind
low Spanish Indigo Spires Sil
ple Rain Mealy Wild Bog Sho
Clary Mexican Roseleaf Wooly
Painted Autumn Rosy Meado
e Littleleaf Fruit Big Blue Purp
e Bee Common Pineapple Cla
d Gentian Indigo Spires Paint
digo Spires Silver Jame Little

Showy White Bee Common
Wooly Cleveland Gentian Ind
Meadow Spanish Indigo Spire
Blue Purple Rain Mealy Wild
neapple Clary Mexican Rosele
ires Painted Autumn Rosy Me
me Littleleaf Fruit Big Blue P
White Bee Common Pineappl
Cleveland Gentian Indigo Spir
panish Indigo Spires Silver Ja
ain Mealy Wild Bog Showy WI
exican Roseleaf Wooly Clevela
tumn Rosy Meadow Spanish

THE SAGE GARDEN

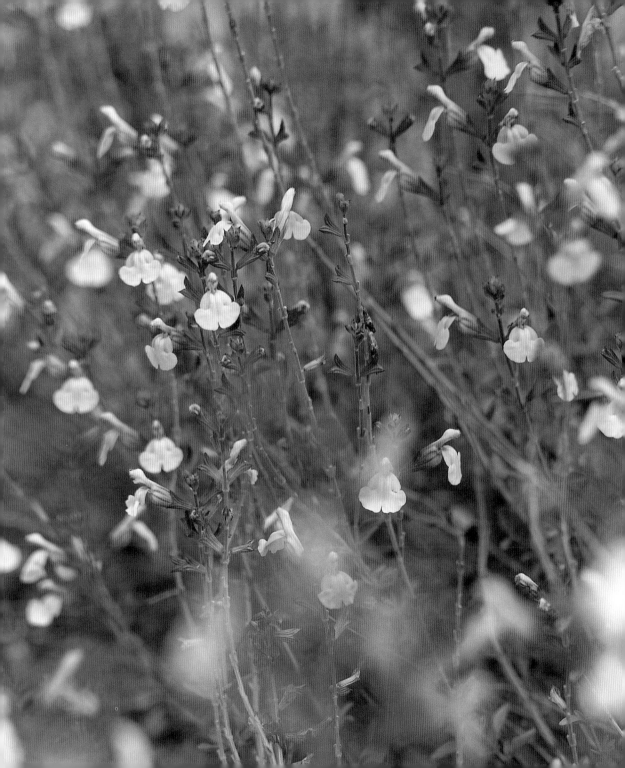

THE SAGE GARDEN

FLOWERS AND FOLIAGE *for* HEALTH AND BEAUTY

by Ann Lovejoy

CHRONICLE BOOKS
SAN FRANCISCO

for BETSY CLEBSCH

wise woman and sage savant *with affection, admiration, and deep respect*

Library of Congress Cataloging-in-Publication Data:
Lovejoy, Ann, 1951–
THE SAGE GARDEN: FLOWERS AND FOLIAGE *for* HEALTH AND BEAUTY by Ann Lovejoy.
p. cm.
ISBN: 0-8118-2758-5
1. Salvia. 2. Salvia—Therapeutic use. I. Title.
SB413.S22 L68 2000   635.9—3396—DC21   00-057091

Printed in Hong Kong

Designed by Frances Baca

Distributed in Canada by Raincoast Books
9050 Shaughnessy Street
Vancouver, British Columbia V6P 6E5

10 9 8 7 6 5 4 3 2 1

Chronicle Books LLC
85 Second Street
San Francisco, California 94105

www.chroniclebooks.com

The publisher's warmest thanks go out to Eric Schulz and Elaine Sedlack at Berkeley Botanical Gardens, and Jeanne Coria and Don Mahoney at Strybing Arboretum for generously providing consultation and salvia identification.

Grey and Ethel would like to extend their very special thanks to Betsy and John Cutler for the generous use of their home, Peter Scott for his location expertise, Elizabeth Glass for her fabulous assisting and location hunting, and Sylvia Roberts for her attention to detail and help in the gardens.

table *of* contents

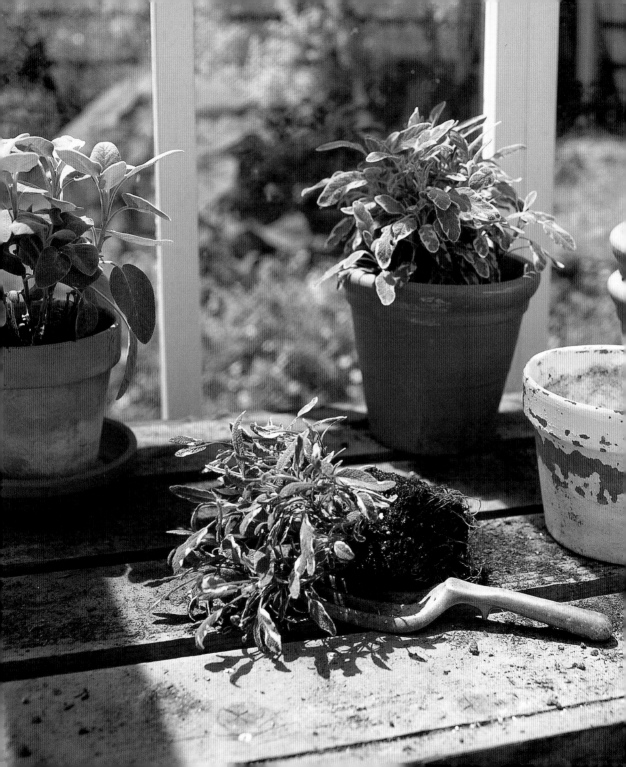

What is sage?

Ask gardeners or cooks in almost any country in the world and they will answer without hesitation. However, the answers you get may vary greatly, for many sages have served many cultures in many ways since time out of mind. Long before history was recorded, nomadic peoples from China to America's Southwest burned sages in spiritual ceremonies, as ashes found in prehistorically painted caves attest. For millennia, sages have been valued for sacred rituals, folk remedies, healing, and culinary uses everywhere they occur in nature. This connection with the sacred goes deep into the murk of prerecorded human history but is traceable to the potent natural oils that permeate so many of the sage species. Both foliage and flowers may be scented, though in some sages, the scent of dried foliage is generally more pleasing than that of the fresh leaves. Indeed, though some sages are commonly described as perfumed, others have a rougher, more complex scent that is too strong or coarse for some tastes. Sage's position in human culture has a curious commonality, despite differences of species or geographical distribution. As evidence of this, consider that the words *save, salvage, salvation, sage,* and the botanical name *Salvia* all share both the common Latin root word *salvare,* "to save," as well as *salvus,* "whole," "safe," and "healthy."

Since ancient times, sage has been associated with at the least the restoration of health and, in many cases, the healing of body, mind, and spirit. In cultures as diverse as those of classical Greece or ancient Asia and the native tribal traditions of Central and North America we find strong historical links between healing ceremonies and native salvias.

Nearly all of sage's traditional associations are similarly wholesome, for the entire family is considered to have healing properties of one kind or another. Sage has historically been associated with gods and goddesses of wisdom, such as Apollo and his sister, Athena. Both of these concepts are reflected in our daily language when we seek for sage advice, when we refer to wise elders as sages, and when we offer each other our salutations (wishes for good health). *Salve,* or "good health," is an ancient Roman greeting still in use today, while French folks toast each other with *Salut,* meaning "to your health," and both languages use the word *sage* to mean wise or philosophically profound. Even in South and Central America, where the tropical sages flourish under the dense canopy of rainforest, sages have been (and still are) used both medicinally and in sacred rituals, and the many names for sage plants are also used to indicate wisdom or healing.

THE SAGE GARDEN Today, we are as apt to grow sages for their ornamental qualities as for their culinary and healing properties. Our introduction to the family is equally likely to be through brilliant bedding sages as by way of that savory kitchen workhorse, culinary sage. Gardeners looking for long-blooming, easygoing plants that will contribute to bed and border over many months without fuss often find themselves developing a sage collection almost by accident. That's because the family as a whole is flexible, adaptive, and cooperative, making them terrific candidates for today's easy-care gardens.

Salvias are so varied as a species that there is literally a plant for almost any place. Dryland sages will appreciate the arid, stony ground along a driveway or parking strip. They also revel in the sometimes harsh reflected heat along a poolside patio. These long bloomers are perfect for anyone who wants to limit water use, whether in desert, chaparral, or high plains gardens.

Those who lack full sun can still grow a wide range of salvias, since many salvias (including dramatic, semitropical understory beauties) will thrive in filtered shade and ordinary garden soil. Bountiful bedding salvias can brighten borders or windowboxes, while larger border beauties look majestic in outsized pots and containers. Though their pungent scents make them unsuitable as cut fresh flowers, several salvias dry well and are prized for flower crafts of many kinds.

When we begin to explore the sage clan, we discover that sages come in an enormous variety of color, size, shape, and kind. The sage clan contains some 900 recognized species of perennial, biennial, and annual herbs as well as shrubs and subshrubs. With representatives on every continent, the sages are classified as cosmopolitan, citizens of the world. It's not surprising that such a well-traveled group would demonstrate its adaptability by displaying a significant variety of form. Thus, we find sages with simple rounded foliage and others with divided or deeply lobed leaves that may be velvety or glossy, matte or leathery. Some sage leaves are tiny and fine textured, while others are coarse and so boldly sized as to appear tropical (which indeed, some of them are).

However varied the foliage, all sages have similar flowers in any color you like, from white to black and nearly every shade in between. Colorists will revel in the palest lavenders, yellows, and pinks, hot corals and reds, and rich blues and purples. No matter what the shade or tint, sage flowers always have tubular or funnel-shaped necks and flaring lips. If you grow some of their relatives in the enormous *Lamiaceae* clan (sage cousins include mint, lemon balm, hyssop, lavender, thyme, horehound, and catmint), you may see a familial likeness between sage flowers and those of many of their kin. In addition, sages often boast floral bracts (specialized leaves that surround buds and flowers) that may be even more colorful and showy than the flowers.

Since the distribution of this great family is worldwide, there is literally a sage for every garden. Historically, a mere few dozen sages have been widely grown, chiefly for medicinal and culinary uses. As interest in ornamental gardening has grown around the world, so has the gardener's appetite for beautiful sages. Modern gardeners can choose among dozens of handsome sages that brighten beds and borders, blooming in steady succession from spring through autumn.

If you love color, this may be the perfect family for your garden. As mentioned, sages flower in a full range of colors and over a long period of time, offering colorists generous quantities of living pigment with which to paint their garden vignettes. If you have a sunny garden with good drainage, you can find a sage in nearly any tint you need to complete your favorite color scheme. In addition, sages of many kinds offer a double color harvest in the form of "flying flowers": butterflies, hummingbirds, and native bees, all of which delight in sage nectar. Shady gardens offer fewer opportunities to explore the sage family, yet gardeners in warm climates will find great pleasure in growing tropical understory sages like the gorgeous showboat called 'Limelight'.

Unlike most of their sun-loving cousins, these Central and South American understory sages prefer light or dappled shade and moister soils and may also need shelter from strong winds that can shatter their brittle branchwork. Until recently, tender perennials have been considered as only useful in the very warmest climates. These days, adventurous gardeners all over the country are growing tropical and semitropical plants as colorful summer annuals. Even if you live in a harsh climate where tender sages must be treated as annuals, you will find that they reward moderate care with abundant bloom.

Traditional bedding sages include some tender perennials as well as true annuals. These short-lived plants bloom with abandon almost anywhere, offering long-lasting flowers that double as cut flowers for the table. Ornamental border sages, long grown in England, offer American gardeners plenty of scope. Colorists can build drama by partnering deep-toned sages like 'Indigo' and 'Purple Rain' with golden foliage or clean white flowers. Those who find the most magic in softer tints and tones can create an old-fashioned garden look with a sea of painted sage in shades of pink and blue, white and rose, lavender and purple, using the 'Claryssa' series as a base for a flurry of cottage flowers.

Statuesque white Turkish sage (*Salvia sclarea 'Turkestanica'*) has the architectural strength to match bold sheaves of grasses and tall prairie plants. Dazzling 'Sizzler Series' annual sages (*S. splendens*) will lace the garden with floral fireworks, bringing volcanic shades of flame and sunset to your tropicalismo border or patio containers. An hour or two spent browsing through garden catalogs will reveal that dozens of sage species and over a hundred named forms are widely available from nurseries and seed sources.

While most popular garden sages are considered purely ornamental, the sturdy band I call "the sages of service" continue to be grown as much for their practical uses as for their good looks. Most of these hail from Europe, where they have long enjoyed a wide range of traditional uses, from culinary to comfort and the curative. Sage leaves flavor hundreds of recipes, from teas and tisanes to soups and stuffings. Extracts of sage flowers are used to treat eye conditions, soften rough skin, and add a subtle, healing fragrance to bath salts. Sage foliage is used to soothe sore throats and digestive troubles, to moderate menses, and even to brew an herbal beer that puts strong men under the table.

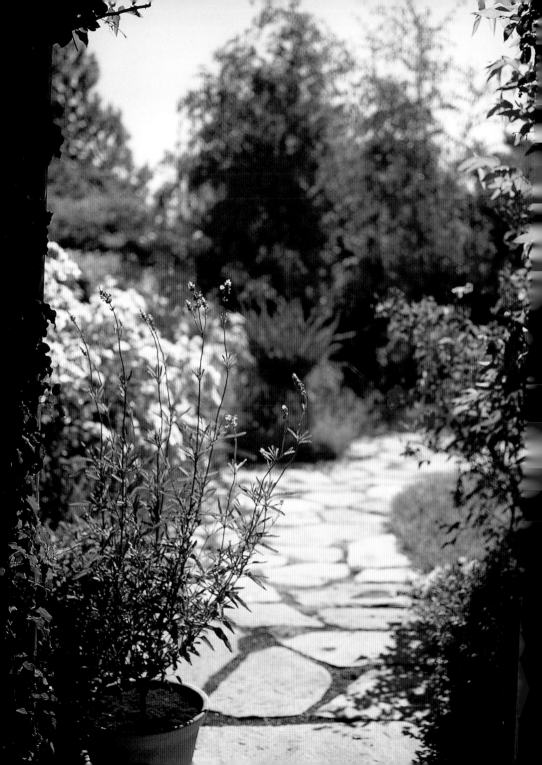

FINDING THE RIGHT SAGE Gardeners who want to explore this fascinating family may find themselves a bit bewildered by its sheer largess. With so many sages from which to choose, how do you go about finding the right one for each site and setting? To simplify your search, chapters 1 through 6 present you with profiles and specific growing tips for sages of certain kinds and purposes. We'll begin with the most adaptable sages, those that grow readily almost anywhere. In chapter 1, you'll meet the meadow sages, a carefree group of annuals and short-lived perennials that will happily decorate bed and border and can also successfully compete in wild or meadow gardens. You'll also be introduced to the "critter collection," sages that act like magnets for bees, birds, and butterflies. Most sages are appealing to all three, but the sages profiled here are particularly irresistible, making them excellent candidates for those who love butterfly gardens or want to encourage hummingbirds to make themselves at home in the garden.

Chapter 2 presents classic border and bedding beauties, plants that reliably produce over a long period in a wide range of garden settings. Some of these species have numerous named forms while others have only one, but all earn star status with companionable manners (they are not greedy or difficult) as well as solid good looks. The bedding sages are hard workers that flower with great goodwill, performing cheerfully even under difficult conditions and rewarding moderate care with an immoderately generous response.

Gardeners who want to limit water use and those who have little water at their disposal (perhaps gardening near or in desert or chaparral environments) will find an enticing palette of plants in chapter 3. Indeed, the dry-country sages give of their best where excess summer water can be avoided. This makes them excellent candidates for xeriscaping (gardening with little or no supplemental water) as well as for gardening in or near desert areas. Wherever autumns are mild and Indian summers common, the late bloomers profiled will bring weeks or even months of color that persists well past Labor Day.

The second half of the book offers plant profiles and growing tips for traditional culinary sages (chapter 4) and the more recently introduced scented sages (chapter 5), which can be used in fruit salads and iced teas as well as potpourri and herbal concoctions. Chapter 6 is filled with recipes for cooking and crafting with these sages of service. The closing lists of sources and resources and books for further reading will help you locate and learn more about the sages that intrigue you. A detailed map and index will help you quickly locate topics of interest.

As you browse the chapters, you'll learn how to dry sages for crafts and culinary uses and how to use your harvest, fresh or dried, in delicious foods, from sage-roasted chicken with a crackling, golden herb-stuffed skin to refreshingly sweet sorbets flavored with fruit sage. You'll find recipes for sage hand lotion and bath herb bags as well as a mild sage and rosemary shampoo that will bring gloss to the driest hair. (I can personally attest to this, since I work outside all the time and my hair gets dry and sun bleached. The shampoo recipe offered here has made my hair more manageable than it's been in years.)

Every chapter also includes information on how to make more of each particular group of sages, whether through division, by taking cuttings, or by saving your own seed. Each plant profile also contains specific directions and cultural tips that will help you succeed with that individual sage. Though many sages have a preference for sun and good drainage, the precise details of their care can vary considerably. Knowing how to please the sages you choose can mean the difference between effortless enjoyment and continual frustration. For instance, a plant that does not want mulch and manure can be killed by "kindness," while a reputed "easy grower" may need coddling in certain climates during the first year before reaching total independence in maturity.

I hope this book will encourage you to try growing some of these remarkable plants in your own garden. Though we will look closely at only a few dozen sages, this necessarily abbreviated sampler will introduce you to some of the stars of the sage species, including both the most useful and the most glamorous kinds. As you read through these pages, take time to stop and try some of the recipes, whether for teas or tisanes, hand lotion or hair rinse, shampoo or smudges. As you become familiar with the properties and fragrances of each kind of sage, you'll find yourself adapting and altering the recipes to suit your own taste or nose. Gardens bring us joy just by being, but when we can also use our plants in our daily life, gathering and preparing them adds another dimension of pleasure and refreshment to gardening, allowing it to sustain our bodies as well as our spirits. To your health!

ANN LOVEJOY *summer 2000*

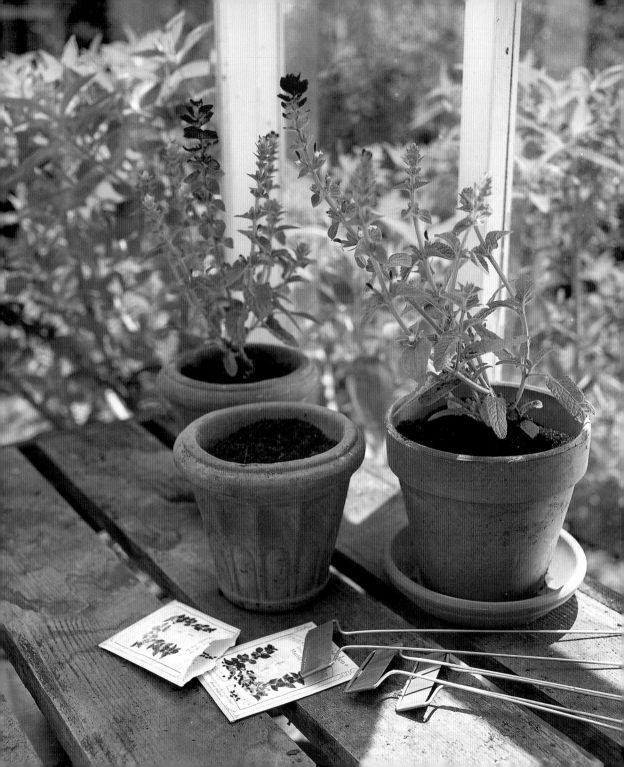

1

meadow sages

Meadow Sage *Salvia pratensis*
Painted Sage *S. viridis (syn. S. horminum)*
Wild Sage *S. x sylvestris group*

vibrant

For most gardeners, meadow sages are among the easiest perennials to please. Native to open meadows in various parts of the world, they grow happily when interwoven with grasses, bulbs, and other perennials. Almost any well-drained soil is acceptable to meadow sages, and they will bring height and color to an uninteresting carpet of ground covers or undemandingly brighten a difficult corner. Not surprisingly, meadow sages can also hold their own in meadow, prairie, or wild gardens, where competition for nutrients can be determined.

This adaptable quality makes them perfect for mixed-border placement, where their willowy stems can intertwine companionably with neighbors like shrub roses and border spiraeas. Depending partly on their provenance and species and partly on local conditions, meadow sages may be annual, biennial, or short-lived perennials.

S. pratensis is one of Britain's few native sages, and selected forms have been grown for centuries. It is also popular in North America, where it makes itself at home without becoming a nuisance. At one time, this easygoing sage was mistakenly banned as an invasive weed in California, but better research established that a different species (*S. virgata*) was the culprit. Redeemed, *S. pratensis* is once again a valued garden plant, particularly where soils are less than ideal.

S. viridis is one of very few true annual sages in cultivation (many others act like annuals if they don't like a garden or get too cold). Found in open meadows from southern Europe into North Africa and western Asia, painted, or paper, sage was grown in England by the 1600s. The popularity of this mildly scented and flavored herb as a culinary flavoring shows how limited the cuisine of the time was.

The group currently clustered as *Salvia x sylvestris* is viewed in several ways. Some experts consider it to encompass a number of natural hybrids (interspecies crosses that occur in natural settings) as well as deliberate crosses and selections made by gardeners. Others define it as any cross, deliberate or natural, between two specific parents (*S. nemorosa* and *S. pratense*). Still others (including Betsy Clebsch, the North American salvia expert) consider *S. sylvestris* to be a highly variable species that has produced many excellent garden forms.

However classified, these once-wild meadow sages are all adaptable plants that grow well in a variety of garden settings. Over many years of cultivation in England and Europe, each species or group has been improved through steady selection and roguing out of unworthy plants. As a result, named selections and garden forms are considerably more showy than their wild relatives. Here are profiles of three great groups of good-looking, hardworking meadow sages that can serve your garden without requiring perfect conditions or coddling.

Meadow Sage *Salvia pratensis* ZONE 3

Meadow sage is a handsome, long-blooming natural beauty with large, coarse foliage and showy spires of bloom. Grown in borders, the generous flower spikes may exceed 3 feet in height, making a solid contribution to careful color compositions. The quilted, deep green foliage may be as much as 6 inches long at the base. The leaves taper as they continue up the bloom stalks, each of which is tipped with purple or blue flowers in long, arching swags. When grown from seed, you may also find plants with rose, pink, or white flowers, but these will be less common.

MEADOW SAGE IN THE GARDEN Among the hardiest of perennials, meadow sage tolerates a wide range of site and cultural conditions. Most forms are easy to please as long as you can provide nutritious but well-drained soil and plenty of sunshine. When given overly rich soil, however, this wildling may dwindle after a few years or may even act like a biennial, blooming in its second year and then dying. This behavior is especially common in heavy clay soils where winters are wet. Sharp drainage and raised beds are advisable in such situations.

Shapely, colorful, and long blooming, meadow sages are attractive border plants and are also a valuable source of cut flowers. In hot climates, meadow sage may flower for a month in late spring, repeating from late summer into autumn if deadheaded (the first flowers are removed as they fade, with the stems cut close to the basal rosette). This second flowering may not occur if the plants become too dry. Where summers are cool, meadow sage blooms in continual spurts from early summer into fall and may linger into winter where the climate is especially mild.

PLEASING PARTNERSHIPS Meadow sage is an upstanding border beauty that has presence in or out of flower, so it looks better with handsome, architectural companions rather than billowy fluff. Try pairing it with arching grasses such as blue-green oat grass (*Helictotrichon sempervirens*) or upright, airy sheaves of golden oat grass (*Briza media*). Like many of its kin, meadow sage also consorts well with evergreen herbs such as rosemary and lavender.

NAMED FORMS OF MEADOW SAGE Meadow sages are more common in England than in the U.S., but more are appearing here each year. Most can be reliably grown from seed, though seedlings may vary in form and color. If you notice an unusually good-looking seedling, perhaps with extra large or showy flowers, save seed from it. If it breeds relatively true, you can start a seed strain of your own.

The selected form called *Haematodes* bears especially big flowers in gentle shades of lavender blue. This plant and others very like it are sometimes lumped together as a seed strain called *Haematodes Group,* all of which are large flowered, softly colored, and short lived. This group is considered to be a subspecies by some authorities and may be sold as *S. pratensis ssp. haematoides* in some nurseries.

ALBA
White flowers

ATROVIOLACEA
Violet-blue flowers

BAUMGARTENII
Purple-blue flowers

HAEMATOIDES
Large, soft lavender-blue flowers

LUPINOIDES
Purple to blue flowers on tall spikes (to 2 feet)

MIDSUMMER
Clear sky-blue flowers

ROSEA
Rose to pinky-purple flowers

RUBICUNDA
Rose-red flowers

TENORII
Ocean blue flowers

VARIEGATA
Blue-and-white flowers

Painted Sage *Salvia viridis (S. horminum)* ZONES 7 | 8

Long called *S. horminum,* this cheerful, upright annual sage has recently been reclassified as a subgroup of *S. viridis* and may be found at many nurseries under this revised name. This is one of the ceremonial sages used in classical Greece, and the burned leaves were also used to purify sickrooms in England and Europe during the Middle Ages and until recent times. The colorful bracts are far showier than the tiny flowers, though both honeybees and solitary bees readily find their way to the nectar. Painted sage dries beautifully, and fresh or dried stems are prized by floral arrangers.

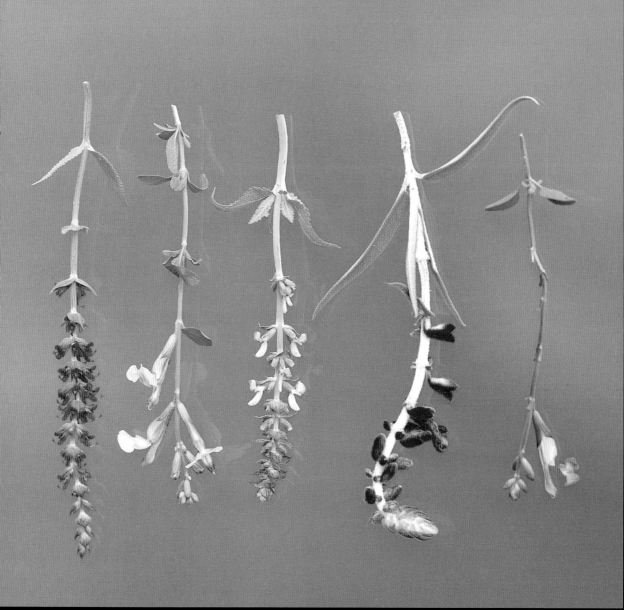

Sage *from left to right*   1 SALVIA X SUPERBA   4 *Salvia leucantha*

PAINTED SAGE IN THE GARDEN Generally grown as a self-sowing annual, painted sage may act as a biennial in warm climates, where the second crop of the season will winter over and bloom the following summer. Painted sage thrives in most gardens but prefers well-drained soils and a sunny setting. In uncrowded beds, this pretty plant self-sows nicely but may be lost in fuller gardens. To be sure of getting seed for next year's crop, gather painted sage when the bracts are dry and beginning to brown off. Store the cut heads in a paper bag with plenty of air. When they are fully dry, shake the bag and the fine seed will be easy to collect.

PLEASING PARTNERSHIPS Like many annuals, painted sage grows with alacrity. Never a pushy plant, painted sage makes an excellent placeholder for new perennials, quickly filling in gaps between youngsters without crowding them. Painted sage's gentle colors blend wonderfully with the varied pinks of old roses, and its shallow roots won't compete with greedy rose roots. It looks best when planted in wide ribbons or drifts, for single plants lack the substance and form needed to stand out in a mixed border.

HARVESTING AND DRYING PAINTED SAGE Painted sage dries very successfully and lasts nicely in dried floral arrangements as long as the flowers are picked when the colorful bracts are well ripened. Soft, flaccid bracts will not dry properly, so hold off harvesting until they feel papery and completely dry to the hand. The flowers themselves should be fully open and at their peak.

To preserve painted sage, pick long-stemmed flower stalks and bundle them in dozens. Snugly fasten the stems together with twine or a rubber band. Dry painted sage upside down and away from the walls or windows. The drying room should be warm, but plants should be hung where they will not receive direct sunlight (a dim attic is perfect). Hang the bundles from a stretched wire or tight string so they get plenty of air from all sides. Once dry (in about a month), painted sage stems can be used in any kind of dried arrangement, wreath, or craft project.

NAMED FORMS OF PAINTED SAGE Seed of named forms runs fairly true, especially in long-established strains, although there may always be a little variation in a crop of seedlings. Keep your eyes open for an especially good form; the forms listed below are mainly garden selections originally made by gardeners with a discerning eye.

ALBA
Clean white bracts

BLUEBEARD
Sky-blue bracts veined in purple

CLARYSSA BLUE
Showy blue bracts veined in black; compact (18 inches)

CLARYSSA MIXED
Showy bracts (white, pink, rose, blue, purple) veined in contrasting colors; compact

CLARYSSA PINK
Showy warm-pink bracts veined in burgundy and green; compact

CLARYSSA WHITE
Showy white bracts veined in green; compact

ROSE BOUQUET
Pink to deep rose bracts

VIOLACEA
Violet bracts veined in purple

Wild Sage *Salvia x sylvestris* group ZONE 5

As mentioned above, this closely related group of species and hybrids is lumped together by several authorities as well as by many gardeners, who can't see many differences between them. Botanists apparently can't either, since there is significant nomenclatorial confusion (or difference of opinion) surrounding this group. Whatever their name, the wild sages make strong, sturdy garden perennials with considerable garden presence. Unselected or straight species plants are rarely if ever seen, but the lovely, easy-to-please garden forms mentioned on the following page are fortunately quite common. Many with Germanic-sounding names ('Mainacht') have been given English versions ('May Night'), and you may see the same plants sold by several names. Most of these were raised in Germany some fifty years ago and are still considered to be among the best of the bunch.

WILD SAGE IN THE GARDEN   The sages in this group are native throughout Europe, and some may be found into Asia Minor. All (including their many garden forms) can be treated similarly, requiring only well-drained garden soil and a sunny setting to produce many weeks of abundant blossom. All are tolerant of dry soils but bloom longest and best with a bit of supplemental water where summers are hot.

As a group, these sages range between 18 inches and 2½ feet in height and may be almost equally wide. Their slim, tapering foliage is clustered densely at the base of each plant, which forms a clump rather than a basal rosette. The usually matte, deeply embossed foliage shades from dull green to gray. While painted sage boasts colorful bracts, these sages offer brightly colored calyces (the calyx is the outer, leafy sheath of a flower). The flowers, which are usually bright purple (though they may be blue or rosy), whorl gaily about their stalks, making slender wands of bloom that may be anywhere from 5 to 10 inches long.

PLEASING PARTNERSHIPS   The rich blues, purples, and violets of this group of sages make them invaluable border plants. Nothing sets off silvers and grays like these luminous sky and water colors, which combine equally well with sunset reds and flame oranges or softer shades of rose, peach, and salmon. The best known of the bunch, 'May Night', has dusky, glowing purple flowers with calyces the color of summer twilight. It makes a splendid counterpoint to regal lilies or silvery lavenders or curry plant (*Helichrysum angustifolium*). The newest introduction, 'Plumosa', is a knockout with generous, fluffy flower heads of rich plum and rose that make a compelling contrast with silvery foliage as well as rosy flowers.

NAMED FORMS OF WILD SAGE

Any may be sold as *S. x sylvestris, S. x superba,* or *S. nemorosa:*

ALBA
White flowers, grayish leaves; 2 feet

EAST FRIESLAND
Dark purple and deep blue bracts

LUBECA
Purple flowers, early blooming; 2 ½ feet

PLUMOSA
Fluffy, plum-colored flowers; 18 inches

SNOW HILL
Fluffy white flowers; to 30 inches

BLUE QUEEN
Purple-blue flowers; compact (18 inches)

KEW GOLD
Old-gold foliage, blue flowers; 2 feet

MAY NIGHT
Midnight blue flowers; to 2 feet

ROSE QUEEN
Gray-green leaves, soft rose flowers, deep rose calyces; compact (18 inches)

VIOLA KLOSE
Warm blue, early blooming; 2 feet

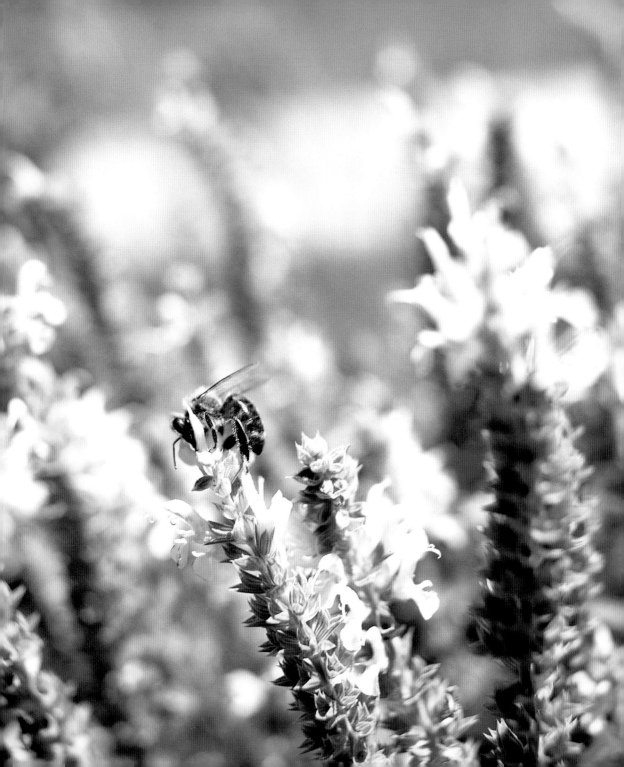

sages *for* bees, butterflies, and hummingbirds

Bee Sage   *Salvia apiana*

Jame Sage   *S. x jamensis*

Woolly Sage   *S. leucantha*

enticing

Today's gardeners often welcome wild creatures into the garden. True, butterflies are more lastingly welcome than raccoons and deer, but the presence of wild things is now valued as an indicator of a healthy environment. When soils and plants are contaminated with garden chemicals, the population of all wildlife is greatly reduced. As we clean up our gardens, we discover that a healthy garden is a happy place to be.

There is a refreshingly joyful quality to gardens that are alive in many respects. Not only are such gardens home to flourishing communities of plants, but they also support a wide spectrum of living creatures. How soothing to the spirit is the gentle hum of busy bees, moving from blossom to blossom with concentrated attention. The sudden flash and flicker of hummingbirds adds a lively blend of movement and color as they perform their aerial battles. Butterflies add balletic grace to the mix, putting on an ever-changing pageant for the observer.

For those who want to draw favorite creatures into their gardens, sages become important members of the welcoming committee. Many butterflies feed avidly upon sage nectar, as do hummingbirds. Like most herbs, sages are highly attractive to nectar- and pollen-collecting insects when in flower. The three sages profiled in this chapter are notably magnetic in their appeal.

North America is rich in native butterflies, from showy painted ladies and swallow-tails to monarchs, all of which will sip happily from most sage blossoms. Some are especially potent; up to thirty-five species of native butterflies visit *Salvia leucantha* and the Jame sages, including great spangled fritillaries, mourning cloaks, and viceroys.

North American bird populations include both migrating and fixed species in ample variety. A naturalistically designed garden can attract dozens of species, since a variety of layered shrubs provide food and shelter. Honeysuckles, roses, sumacs, chokecherries, and other fruiting shrubs will fill the bill nicely.

Flower gardens attract worm lovers like robins, seed eaters such as goldfinches, and nectar drinkers such as hummingbirds, which often hover above sage plants. Anna's and ruby-throated hummers feed eagerly on purple Mexican sage (*S. mexicana*) and blue bog sage (*S. uliginosa*). Any red sage will make hummingbirds happy, including showy sage (*S. splendens*), autumn sage (*S. greggii*), pineapple sage (*S. elegans*), and rosy sage (*S. coccinea*).

Most flowers, fruit, and vegetables are dependent on bees and other insect pollinators for production. For those disappointed in low yields, attracting bees to the garden helps dramatically. In a decade, North American populations of European honeybees have dropped by up to 9o percent. Bees are extremely sensitive to herbicides and pesticides. Once exposed, their immune systems are damaged and they become highly susceptible to many pests and diseases.

Most native bees (such as mason bees and bumblebees) are solitary rather than hiving. As European bees made their way west, these more efficient hiving bees crowded out the less competitive natives. To support all bees, eliminate toxic chemicals in the garden (and anywhere else possible). Next, provide the longest possible bloom period, providing snow crocus, hellebores, and early blooming shrubs in winter and extending autumn bloom with late flowering asters, goldenrods, and salvias.

MAKING WILDLIFE FEEL AT HOME To make gardens safe for wildlife, use nontoxic insecticidal soaps or rinse pests off plants with hose water. Birds also help, since many feed at least partially on insects (hummingbirds eat several times their weight in insects each day). In truth, most insects are beneficial rather than troublesome and a healthy population of beneficial predators helps keep "bad bugs" under control.

To attract wildlife, fill the yard with herbs and flowering shrubs. Plants in variety attract and support creatures in variety. Many will prefer native plants, so blend some in with your border beauties. The longer your bloom season, the richer and healthier your wildlife populations will be, so stretch the garden year with winter-blooming snowdrops and fall-flowering Japanese anemones.

Casual cottage gardens or mixed border gardens offer better cover for wild creatures than formal styles. Cottage gardens mingle edibles with ornamentals, boasting flowers and fruit through much of the year. Mixed borders layer small trees, shrubs, perennials, and ground covers with bulbs and ornamental grasses in natural rather than contrived-looking plantings. Sheltering shrubs such as lilacs, butterfly bushes, and twiggy dogwoods provide resting and nesting spots out of the wind.

A birdbath or small pool pleases birds, and male butterflies will "puddle" for minerals in the damp soil found beneath an actively used birdbath. A sunny site will draw a higher percentage of visitors than a shady one, but a mixture of sun and shade is best of all. Provide all this and you'll find an ever greater parade of bees, birds, and butterflies dancing daily through your garden.

Bee Sage *Salvia apiana* ZONE 8

This California chaparral native is admired for its pungent, penetrating perfume and for the beauty of its tapered, whorling, silvery leaves covered with soft, silken hairs. Long, slender, and neatly creased down their slim middle, the 3- to 4-inch leaves are set on woolly stems tipped by white flowers that are often stippled and speckled with lavender. In the wild, this rangy evergreen shrub may stretch 5 feet in height, often growing leggy over time. The Latin name, *apiana*, means "of bees," so it is not surprising that where bee sage is common, beekeepers take advantage of its allure and set their hives near the bushes in late spring, when they begin to bloom. The honey is often sold as white sage blossom honey and brings the distinctive, almost resinous scent and savor of the glittering foliage to the breakfast table.

BEE SAGE IN THE GARDEN Not picky about soil type, bee sage does demand sharp drainage and full sun. It thrives in difficult, dry spots where ordinary border beauties fail. Lester Rowntree, one of California's ardent naturalists, often said that she lost more California natives to coddling and kindness than to neglect. Her recipe for success with chaparral plants works well for bee sage; in Lester's wide experience, California natives like bee sage were happiest on a sloping, east-facing bank, preferably set among a few rocks. Sage specialist Betsy Clebsch writes that bee sage is particularly beautiful by moonlight, especially if partnered with similarly luminous plants such as artemisias and senecios. To keep bee sage plants compact and shapely, trim back the longest stems by half (or more) after the flowers fade in midsummer.

PLEASING PARTNERSHIPS Garden plants of bee sage make upright mounds of sparkling, silvery foliage that contrast dramatically with dark foliage, whether of New Zealand flax (*Phormium tenax*) or native purple sand cherry (*Prunus x cistena*). Bee sage also looks at home with white Spanish broom (*Cytisus multiflorus*) and the lovely pink- and purple-flowered sterile hybrids like 'Lavender Time' and 'Pink Spot', as well as silky, silver-leaved pineapple broom, *Cytisus battandieri*. To keep butterflies and other critters coming, partner bee sage with a succession of long-blooming penstemons and agastaches as well as late-blooming euphorbias.

NAMED FORMS OF BEE SAGE Though Californian nurseries carry selected forms and hybrids of bee sage, not many have been given names so far. Check nurseries for good garden forms, which tend to be more compact.

VICKI ROMO
Compact hybrid with *S. clevelandii* (3 feet); blue flowers

Jame Sage *Salvia x jamensis* ZONES 7 | 8 | 9

This beautiful new group of sages was discovered near the Mexican village of Jame in the Sierra Madre in the early 1990s and immediately took western gardens by storm. In just a few years, named forms have made their way to nurseries across the States and to England. A natural hybrid of two southwestern species, *S. greggii* and *S. microphylla* (see chapter 3), Jame sage combines the good looks and long-flowering habits of both parents with a wider range of flower colors. Where summers are hot, these compact shrubs reach 3 feet in height and width, though in coastal gardens they may grow considerably larger. In cooler areas, Jame sage may be treated as an annual and will bloom its heart out as a 2-foot plant. The slim stems bear neatly embossed, leathery little leaves of a rich, glossy green and are tipped with short sprays of brilliantly colored flowers that repeat from mid-summer until frost.

JAME SAGE IN THE GARDEN This Mexican bush sage blooms from midsummer into autumn, often continuing into winter where frost is rare. The hybrids are variously hardy, with some surviving zone 7 winters and others vanishing in zone 8. Success seems to depend on soil drainage and accumulated summer heat; in cool, clay-based gardens, these sages are not happy campers. Give them lean, well-drained soil, full sun, and little summer water, and they bloom with vigor and return with zest. Jame sages grow well in containers and may be overwintered in a frost-free garage or greenhouse.

Pleasing partnerships Its wide color range makes Jame sage a useful bedding and border plant. The softer yellow and peachy shades partner beautifully with long-flowering yarrows (*Achillea*) such as 'Moonlight', 'Terra Cotta', and 'Sandstone'; toast-and-tea-colored verbascums such as 'Jackie' and 'Helen Johnson'; and coppery carexes such as *Carex buchananii* and *C. comans* 'Bronze'. Hotter reds and pinks mingle excitingly with purple rain sage (see chapter 2) and carpeting roses in similar shades.

Named forms of Jame sage

CIENEGA DES SOL
Peach and buttery-yellow flowers; 2–3 feet

LA LUNA
Moonlight yellow flowers with sand-colored lips; 2–3 feet

PAT VLASTO
Hot pink flowers, midnight calyces; to 3 feet

RASPBERRY ROYALE
Rich raspberry-sorbet flowers; 18 inches

SAN ISIDRO MOON
Chalky pink flowers, midnight purple calyces; 2–3 feet

SIERRA SAN ANTONIO
Peachy pink flowers with yellow lips; to 3 feet

Woolly Sage *Salvia leucantha* ZONES 8 | 9

Long a favorite bedding and border plant in England, woolly sage is popular with butterfly gardeners for its long and late bloom period. Its white flowers are snugged into purple or violet calyces that gleam like gems amid the fuzzy white stem hairs that deck the long bloom stalks. Young plants boast velvety, gray-green, ribbon-thin leaves that deepen to green with age. Where hardy, woolly sage builds over time into a subshrub with a woody base, and plants may be evergreen where winters are mild. In cooler regions at the edge of its hardiness, it acts as a hardy perennial, dying back to the roots each year, then resprouting from the base in early spring.

WOOLLY SAGE IN THE GARDEN Where hardy, woolly sage is a rapid spreader, its base increasing steadily each year. To increase your stock, simply pull a few rooted stems from the outer portions of your mother plant each spring (fall division is less successful). Established plants bloom from midsummer into early winter or until cut down by frost. To promote long bloom, remove fading flower stems every few weeks and they will quickly be replaced with fresh ones.

Where borderline-hardy, this lovely sage is most persistent when grown in raised beds with gritty, very sharply drained soil, full sun, and excellent air flow. In maritime gardens, it tolerates salt spray and grows well in exposed, windy sites. It prefers lean soils to rich ones, where winter wet may be fatal. Woolly sage grows well in large containers, and dormant plants can be wintered over in a frost-free garage.

PLEASING PARTNERSHIPS Woolly sage looks comfortable with a wide range of drought-tolerant sun lovers, from tall sedums such as 'Autumn Joy' and 'Stardust' to heathers and brooms and low-growing California lilacs (*Ceanothus species*). It also partners well with another delightful sage species, *S. melissodora* (hardy to zone 9), sometimes called the grape-scented sage. This upright sage has gray-green foliage and deep blue flowers with dusky near-black calyces. The flowers appear in succession from late spring into autumn, scenting the garden with a perfume that seems as attractive to bees, butterflies, and hummingbirds as to humans.

NAMED FORMS OF WOOLLY SAGE Though several good color variations get passed from garden to garden, as yet few are formally named though you may find them at nurseries labeled in various ways. Here are the most common:

BLUE FORM
Clear blue flowers, deep blue calyces

MIDNIGHT
Violet flowers, purple calyces

PURPLE VELVET
Purple flowers, purple calyces

WHITE FORM
White flowers, pale lavender calyces

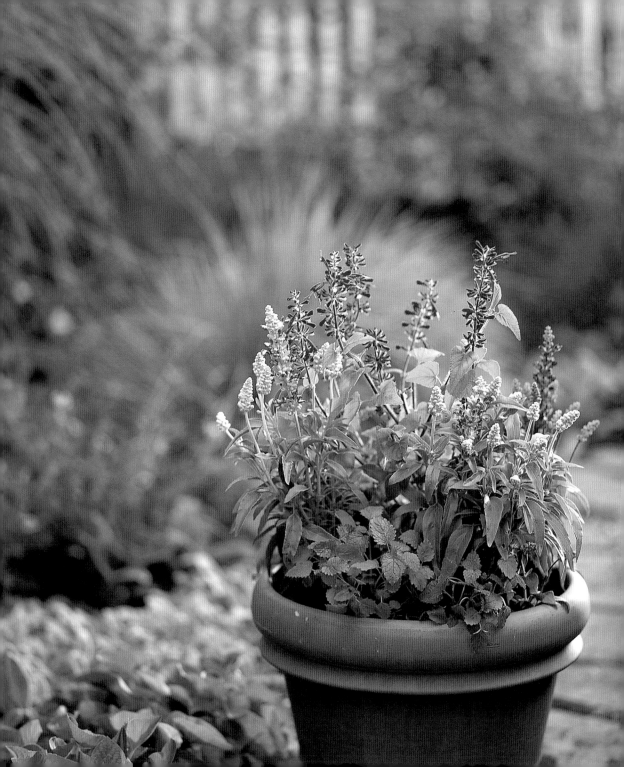

2

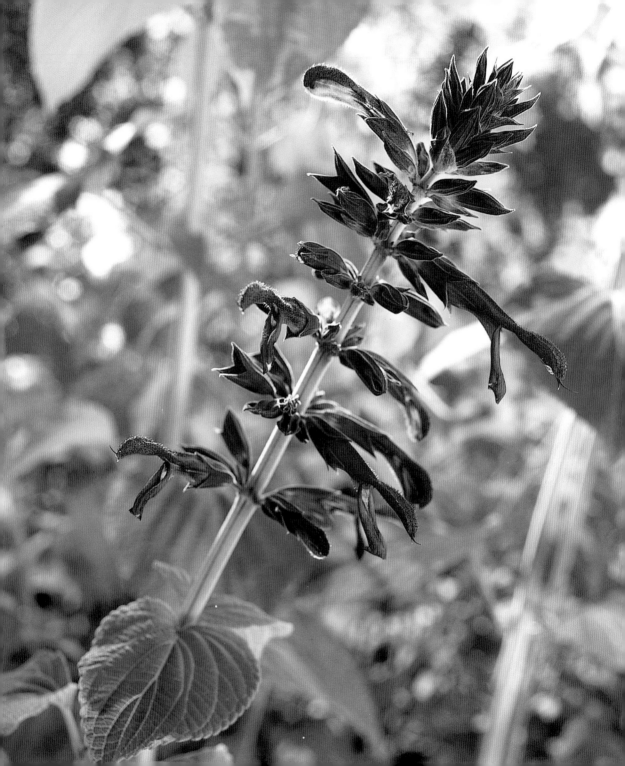

classic border sages

Purple Rain Sage *Salvia verticillata*

Mexican Sage *S. mexicana*

Roseleaf Sage *S. involucrata*

Silver Sage *S. argentea*

dynamic

Selected over the years from among the most ornamental of the sage clan, these choice plants have been improved by generations of gardeners in several countries. These bountiful border beauties share several common characteristics, starting with good architectural form. All have sufficient bulk and adequately sturdy structure to hold their own beside powerfully shaped grasses and border shrubs. Any of these attractive species are terrific choices for important border positions where clean lines and massive displays are desired.

These border sages also offer a prolonged season of abundant bloom (or great looks, in the case of *S. argentea*). Roseleaf sage (*S. involucrata*) may be in flower from May into December in a warm year, and in very mild winters, rosy bracts still unopened in fall may even winter over to open early in spring.

The relatively recent introduction, *S. mexicana*, is already considered indispensable by gardeners who want to attract bees and butterflies to their gardens, because this plant blooms long and hard and the purple-blue flowers are always alive with insects. Its stunning selection, 'Limelight', has enough presence to pull an unstructured border together, and makes a natural centerpiece whenever it's placed amid other plants.

Though 'Purple Rain' can be a slow starter (especially after a cool winter), it will make up for a quiet spring by flowering long and late, often continuing into early winter. The only swan in a family of ducklings, 'Purple Rain' exchanges the lax form and subtle beauties of its parent species for a unique style of its own. Upright, compact, and sturdy, this is the purple salvia of choice for those with smaller gardens. It looks lovely when softening the edge of a pathway and makes a memorable container planting.

Silver sage (*S. argentea*) is not noted for its flowers (though the soft pink blossoms have their admirers). It's claim to fame is fabulous form, sumptuous texture, and a sparkling color matched by few other plants in any palette. Where winters are mild and not excessively wet, silver sage continues to make its mark through the cooler months, when its great leaves reveal a lovely purple-blue sheen beneath their damp silvery fur.

If none of the other border sages profiled here can quite match silver sage for foliar splendor, they can all claim to be at least handsome or even dramatic in leaf. Mexican sage foliage can be slightly gray or downright pewtery, with a soft luster that sets off its jewel-toned purple blossoms to perfection. The velvety leaves of 'Purple Rain' look as if they were stamped from thick felt, then neatly trimmed with pinking shears. These best-of-the-border sages will definitely make their powerful presence felt in your garden compositions.

Purple Rain Sage *Salvia verticillata* ZONE 6

This species is common throughout Europe, where it thrives in all kinds of sites and situations. Modest in manners and looks, it ranges from 1 to 3 feet and can be lax in form. It has produced one stunning garden plant, 'Purple Rain', a compact 2-footer with upright stalks covered in airy, almost starry, blooms. Hardy and long-flowering, this adaptable plant produces waves of deep purple flowers from midsummer into fall.

PURPLE RAIN SAGE IN THE GARDEN   To get the longest and best performance from 'Purple Rain', give it an airy position in full sun. Any good garden soil that offers sharp drainage will do; and though tolerant of drought once established, this plant blooms longest and best when given regular summer water. To keep a long sequence of bloom coming, deadhead spent flower stalks regularly. To protect it from frost, leave the stalks unpruned until spring.

PLEASING PARTNERSHIPS   The deep, dramatic flower color makes 'Purple Rain' sage a marvelous companion for silvery herbs like curry plant (*Helichrysum angustifolia*) and lavenders. It also complements the often hot pinks of old roses as well as the chartreuse of lady's mantle (*Alchemilla mollis*). Shimmering grasses like ponytail grass (*Stipa tenuissima*) and copper *Carex flagellifera* also set off the deep color excitingly, as does the rose-and-purple tall sedum 'Vera Jameson'.

Mexican Sage *Salvia mexicana* ZONE 8

In the wild, Mexican sage is found in variable terrain, so it is not surprising that it comes in many shapes and sizes. Its garden forms are also varied, ranging in height from 3 to 6 feet and in leaf color from gray green to dull green. All are late bloomers that begin to flower in late summer (often August) and continue until frost. Where summers are cool, Mexican sage may bloom too late to be of value to summer gardeners but will be prized by those who want the borders to carry on as long as possible.

MEXICAN SAGE IN THE GARDEN This lusty subtropical sage grows well in light or high shade and will bloom abundantly under tall trees. It takes full morning sun in stride but needs protection from hot afternoon sun in summer. Well-drained soil is a must, especially at the edges of its hardiness range, where wet winters and clay soil can be fatal. In such places, raised beds of gritty soil, well amended with compost, will prove most satisfactory. To keep this long-legged beauty in shape, trim back overwintered stems in spring and shorten again as flowers fade.

PLEASING PARTNERSHIPS Mexican sage is a stunning plant with presence even in its first year, building in time into a billowing, bushy long bloomer that can stop traffic, particularly in its showiest form, 'Limelight'. To make the most of this glamorous form, underplant it with 'Sunfast Chartreuse' coleus and bushy mounds of *Helichrysum petiolare* 'Limelight'.

NAMED FORMS OF MEXICAN SAGE While there are quite a few garden selections of this variable species, only a few are readily found. 'Limelight' is rapidly becoming a must-have border plant; the other three varieties listed below are dazzlers:

COMPTON'S FORM
Purple flowers, near-black calyces;
to 5 feet

LIMELIGHT
Deep purple flowers, lime-green calyces;
to 6 feet

LOLLY JACKSON
Purple-blue flowers;
compact and bushy (to 4 feet)

OCAMPO
Purple flowers; upright (to 7 feet)

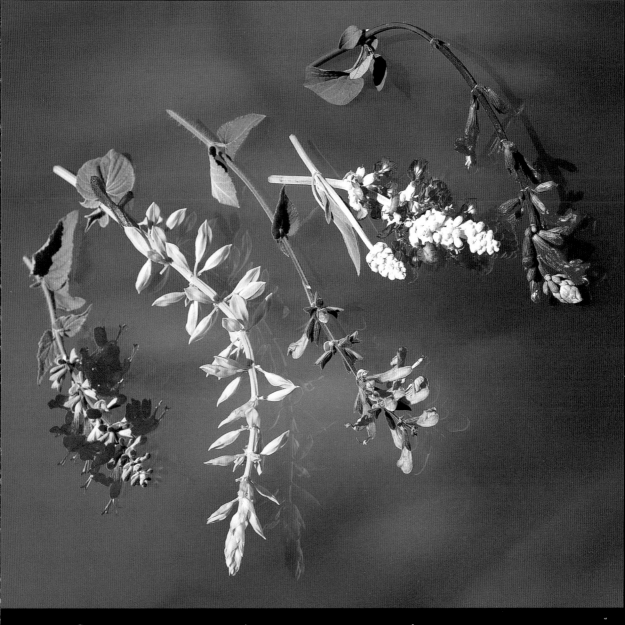

Sage *from left to right*

1 *Salvia coccinea 'Lady in Red'*
LADY IN RED

2 *Salvia mexicana 'Limelight'*
LIMELIGHT

4 *Salvia farinacea 'Strata'*
STRATA

5 *Salvia involucrata 'El Cielo'*
ROSEBUD SAGE

Roseleaf Sage *Salvia involucrata* ZONE 8

In its native Mexico, stands of roseleaf sage are found in the shelter of tall trees. An ever-green shrub in mild climates, it may act like a deciduous shrub or a perennial where winters are cooler. Roseleaf sage flowers from high summer until frost. Named forms are increasingly popular for summer bedding and containers. Roseleaf sage comes easily from spring or summer cuttings. Cut back hard in late spring to promote bushiness.

ROSELEAF SAGE IN THE GARDEN Like other understory sages, roseleaf sage grows well in partial or filtered shade. Where summers are hot, it prefers direct morning sun to blazing afternoon light. However, where summers are cool (in coastal gardens and in the maritime Northwest), roseleaf sage grows best against a warm, south-facing wall. It appre-ciates any good, well-drained garden soil. In dry summers, regular watering increases and prolongs bloom. In the coldest areas, grow roseleaf sage in containers and overwinter in a cool greenhouse.

PLEASING PARTNERSHIPS Big, bold bushes of roseleaf sage look wonderful behind lavender and catmint. In big gardens, I like to put this long bloomer where the reticu-lated bud clusters can be examined close at hand. For a charming vignette, plant roseleaf sage between a red-leaved rose (*Rosa glauca*) and pleated tussocks of lady's mantle (*Alchemilla mollis*).

NAMED FORMS OF ROSELEAF SAGE In England, roseleaf sage forms such as 'Bethellii' have been beloved border beauties for over a century. These days, this Mexican bush sage is coming into its own again with new forms like 'Mulberry Jam'.

BETHELLII
Rose red flowers (3–5 feet)

EL CIELO
Airy, hot pink flowers (5–6 feet)

FRED BOUTIN
Purple-pink flowers, compact (3–4 feet)

HADSPEN
Airy, warm rose flowers, compact (3–5 feet)

MULBERRY JAM
Warm pink flowers, purple calyces, compact (4 feet)

Silver Sage *Salvia argentea* ZONE 5

This outstanding foliage plant grows wild in southern Europe, where its fat, felted rosettes can be seen in rugged Mediterranean meadows. Well-grown plants may reach 3 feet in width, making a wide, spreading skirt of basal leaves that can be over a foot long. The thick, almost succulent leaves are woolly with silken hairs that reflect light, making silver sage a shining star in the border. There are no named or selected forms.

SILVER SAGE IN THE GARDEN Like most hairy, silvery plants, silver sage prefers full sun and excellent drainage and grows best where air circulation is constant. The thick leaves are extremely attractive to slugs and snails, so beginning in late winter an ecologically friendly slug deterrent such as Sluggo should be tucked beneath the rosette periodically. Silver sage thrives in well-amended border soils that drain well and does best in raised beds where native soils are heavy. If allowed to bloom, silver sage often acts like a biennial. To keep this short-lived perennial around, remove the 3-foot flower stalks either before or immediately after bloom. Since the dull white or pale pink flowers are insignificant, this is no great loss; the real attraction lies in the lovely leaves, which are worthy of a conspicuous, front-of-the-border position.

PLEASING PARTNERSHIPS Almost anything looks great with the wide, silken rosettes of silver sage. In winter, the big leaves have the look of blue-gray cabbages with a delicate, pearlescent luster. Pair silver sage with silver-green fountains of evergreen *Carex buchananii* 'Viridis' and mats of creeping thyme or lacy sprawls of *Artemisia stelleriana* 'Silver Brocade' for a delicious vignette that persists all winter. In summer, a backdrop of blue rue (*Ruta graveolens* 'Blue Beauty') and mounds of plum-colored *Euphorbia dulcis* 'Chameleon' make silver sage a knockout.

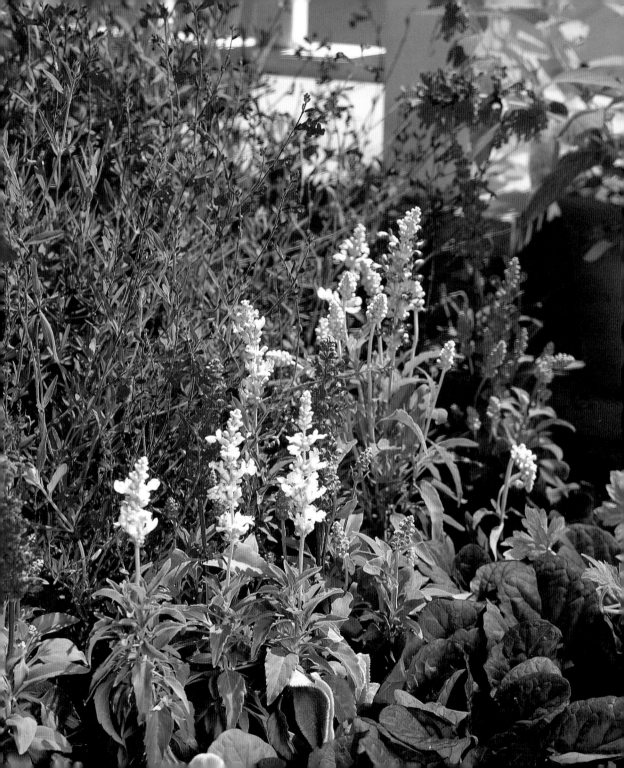

bedding sages

Rosy Sage *Salvia coccinea*
Mealy Sage *S. farinacea*
Showy Sage *S. splendens*

brilliant

Though perennial in the warmest climates, the brilliant, bountiful bedding sages are prized throughout England, Europe, and North America as ardent, long-blooming annuals that perform unflaggingly almost anywhere. In recent years, the popular trend for growing half-hardy or tender perennials has encouraged many cool-region gardeners to erect small greenhouses. In such a sheltered and heated spot, all of these engaging bedders can sail through winter unscathed.

Like many salvias, these willing species adapt well to the restrictions of container life, particularly when grouped in oversized pots or generous planting boxes. If very large planters are used, avoid peat-based soil mixtures, which dry out rapidly and are very hard to rewet. Should they ever dry out, water will tend to run down between the pot side and the soil, leaving the soil completely dry.

Even light soil mixes may become compacted in large containers. To avoid "sour soil," a common condition in poorly oxygenated soils, blend some activated charcoal into the soil before planting. A cupful of charcoal per cubic foot of soil (one medium bag) is plenty. If your garden center does not carry horticultural charcoal, the kind used for fish filters works just as well.

To reduce the frequency of watering without stressing your plants, you may also want to mix in some water-holding crystals (hydrophyllic polymers). These fascinating substances can absorb many times their own weight in water. As they do so, they alter in appearance, swelling up until they look like pieces of soft ice. These water-filled globs act as reservoirs for thirsty plant roots. To be effective, they belong only in the bottom two-thirds of each container. Water-holders placed near the surface of the soil encourage shallow roots that dry out quickly and fail to anchor plants properly.

As long as you are able to keep them well watered, the best of the bedders will bloom for months on end. Since container-grown plants are unable to reach true soil to replenish nutrients, they are dependent on you for all their needs. While bedding sages planted in good garden soil seldom require supplemental feeding, pot plants definitely will. Each time we water a pot, we are leaching out nutrients, so it's crucial to replace them often.

The most effective programs involve frequent light feedings. In general, it's best to dilute fertilizers to half the recommended strength to avoid burning pot-bound roots. As with any fertilizer application, nutritional waterings should always be given after regular watering so both soil and plant roots are damp. This, too, helps to prevent delicate feeder roots from burning.

Each of the three species profiled in this chapter are available in a rich variety of color forms. Every year, new introductions appear, often demonstrating important breaks in plant breeding. Hot oranges and delicate pinks, creamy salmons and sizzling corals extend the usual salvia color range dramatically. Each season, the reds get richer and the purples grow more regal. Some of the showiest newest forms are beautifully bicolored, with deep-toned bracts setting off paler flowers to perfection. Every summer, our choices are more enticing. How can we choose? For my part, when faced with tough decisions, I simply buy them all, placing any extras into pots. Okay, sometimes this means I then need to buy more pots, but that's how the garden grows.

Rosy Sage *Salvia coccinea* SOME FORMS PERENNIAL IN ZONES 9 | 10

Cheerful patches of rosy sage are found throughout much of South America. The species ranges from 2 to 4 feet in height and girth, and many color variations are found in nature. Bedding forms are generally more compact and floriferous, and most bloom through summer into fall. The glossy, rich green leaves are deeply veined, fuzzed with silver-gray beneath, and shaped like elongated hearts.

ROSY SAGE IN THE GARDEN Where hardy, rosy sage prefers well-drained soils. When grown as a bedding annual, it appreciates good garden soil, well amended with compost and an airy mulch of shredded leaves (do not mulch with shredded bark, however). Though a heavy bloomer by nature, it produces best when given regular summer water. If deadheaded as flowers fade, rosy sage will produce an ongoing sequence of flowers from midsummer until cut down by frost. In containers, weekly doses of plant food (at half the suggested strength) will keep the flowers coming steadily all season.

PLEASING PARTNERSHIPS Tall bursts of scarlet-flowered rosy sage make dramatic counterpoints to the large, tropical-looking foliage of hardy cannas and red or green bananas. The softer, ice cream pinks of 'Cherry Blossom' and 'Brenthurst' are beautifully set off by a froth of tiny-leaved silver-gray *Helichrysum microphylla* and peachy daylilies like 'Pink Puff'. White forms look smashing in front of a haze of Russian sage (*Perovskia atriplicifolia*), with masses of filmy, steel wool–colored *Artemisia canescens* at their lovely feet.

NAMED FORMS OF ROSY SAGE

BRENTHURST
Pale pink, large flowers; 2–3 feet

CHERRY BLOSSOM
Cream and soft salmon-pink flowers; 2 feet

LACTEA
White flowers; to 3 feet

LADY IN RED
Scarlet flowers; compact (18 inches)

SNOW BIRD
White flowers, heavy bloomer; to 3 feet

Mealy Sage *Salvia farinacea* ZONE 9

Wild forms of mealy sage grow tall and rangy, making upright plants that may reach 4 feet in height. In tropical climates, mealy sage is an evergreen shrub. At the edges of its hardiness range, it may act as a deciduous shrub or as a perennial. Slim, tapering, glossy green leaves cover long stems that are tipped with blue, purple, or occasionally white flowers. Woolly white calyces give the plant the flour-dusted look that led to its botanical name (*farina* means "flour" in Latin).

MEALY SAGE IN THE GARDEN   In the warmest areas where it persists as an evergreen, mealy sage prefers well-drained soils. To keep this long-blooming sage happy as an annual, give it a sunny spot in rich soil that has been generously amended with compost, and water it weekly during dry spells. Deadheading spent flowers stimulates the production of new ones, which appear more readily when these plants are fertilized at least monthly. If grown in containers, fertilize weekly, using half the suggested amount of plant food, for best performance. Where summers are warm, mealy sage may reach 2 feet or more. In cooler areas, the same plant may only reach 15 or 18 inches but will bloom just as luxuriantly if well fed.

PLEASING PARTNERSHIPS   The clean blues of mealy sage harmonize with almost anything, making these among the easiest plants to place. Sandwich silvery 'Strata' between the black, almost petal-less blossoms of *Rudbeckia* 'Black Beauty' and sprawls of hardy *Geranium x* 'Chocolate Candy', with chocolate leaves and soft pink flowers. Set 'White Porcelain' behind clumps of icy 'Frosty Morning' sedum, with a clump of airy maiden grass, *Miscanthus sinensis* 'Graziella', tucked behind. Any mealy sage makes a lovely underplanting for pink, white, or yellow roses, and all mingle well with short, tufting blue grasses such as *Festuca ovina* 'Sea Urchin'.

BLUE BEDDER
Clear ocean-blue flowers; 18 inches to 2 feet

CIRRUS
Icy white flowers; 2–14 inches

DELFT
China-blue flowers; 18 inches to 2 feet

PORCELAIN
Deep blue flowers; 18 inches to 2 feet

STRATA
Silvery buds, sky-blue flowers;
14 inches to 2 feet

VICTORIA
Deep purple-blue flowers;
18 inches to 2 feet

WHITE PORCELAIN
White flowers with silvery buds;
18 inches to 2 feet

Showy Sage *Salvia splendens* ZONE 10

This Brazilian beauty adapts well to less tropical situations, but where it is grown as a hardy plant, it does best when given the warm, sheltered, and moist conditions it enjoys at home. In the wild, showy sage is an evergreen shrub that prefers a shaded, understory setting.

SHOWY SAGE IN THE GARDEN Showy sage ranks among the world's most popular bedding plants. To get the most from this versatile beauty, give it a rich, moisture-retentive soil and a light mulch of aged compost. It will bloom longest and best if offered plenty of water and regular feeding (twice monthly, but at half the suggested strength). Where hardy (zone 10), showy sage prefers well-drained soil and a leaner diet. In warm gardens it may sow itself about a bit, though it never becomes a nuisance. The old Dutch form 'Van Houttei' makes an evergreen shrub where hardy and requires partial shade, well-drained soil, and shelter from wind.

PLEASING PARTNERSHIPS These quintessential bedding sages are most pleasing when used with flair and imagination. Their uniformity of size and habit make them perfect for carpet bedding in patterns, but they can also be interplanted with small clumping grasses, tall and sprawling sedums, and creeping thymes to make a lively and colorful matrix. Try mixing rich purple 'Salsa' sages with golden feverfew (*Tanacetum parthenium* 'Aureum') and Carex comans 'Bronze', or blend brilliant ribbons of 'Orange Zest' into the same company for a totally different effect. Pack lively 'Salsa' and 'Sizzler' forms into containers with foliage plants such as 'Sunfast Series' coleus in rich chartreuse and burgundy, tumbles of golden creeping Jenny (*Lysimachia nummularia* 'Aurea'), and the 'Licorice' Series of velvet-leaved everlastings (*Helichrysum petiolare*).

NAMED FORMS OF SHOWY SAGE Showy sage is often sold in color mixtures like the new 'Spice of Life'. This seed strain produces a sumptuous run of smoky pastels in muted but potent shades of salmon, mauve, rose, and pink as well as burgundy, purple, and white on compact plants 12 inches tall. Color mixtures can be grown in flats or nursery beds and placed in the garden as the flower colors reveal themselves. Some, like the 'Sizzler Series', are becoming available as single colors as well as mixtures.

BLAZE OF FIRE
Scarlet flowers, early; 12 inches

RED ARROWS
Clear red flowers; upright (10–12 inches)

SIZZLER BURGUNDY
Smoky wine-red flowers; 10–12 inches

VAN HOUTTEI
Shrubby, deep red flowers, chartreuse
foliage; 3–5 feet

ORANGE ZEST
Soft orange flowers; uniform (12 inches)

SALSA SERIES
Vivid colors and pastels; compact (8–12 inches)

SPLENDIDISSIMA
Hot orange flowers, long spikes (8–12 inches)

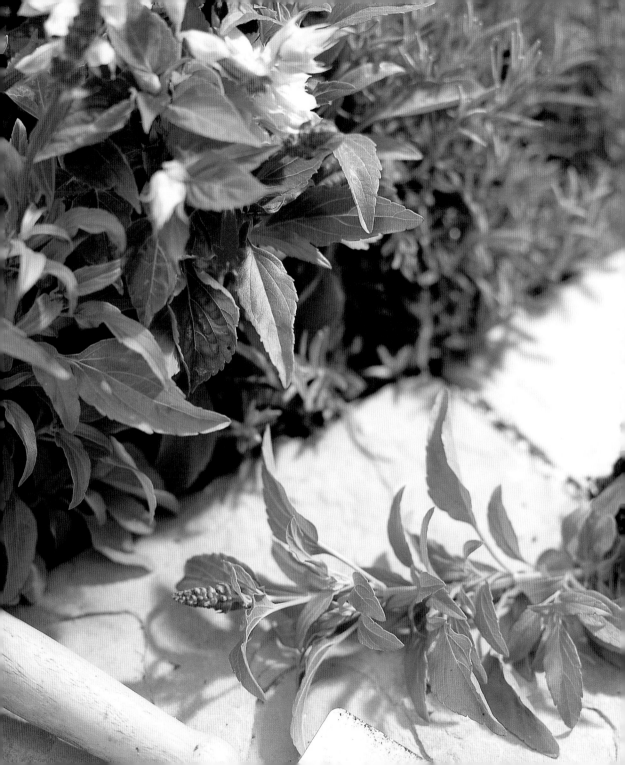

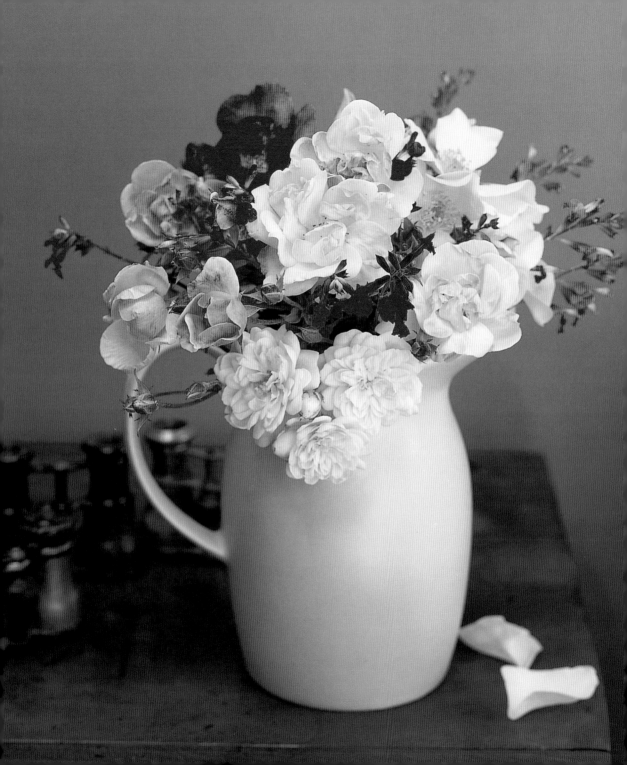

Littleleaf Sage

Autumn Sage

Gentian Sage

White Sage

Big Blue Sage

Bog Sage

Indigo Spires Sage

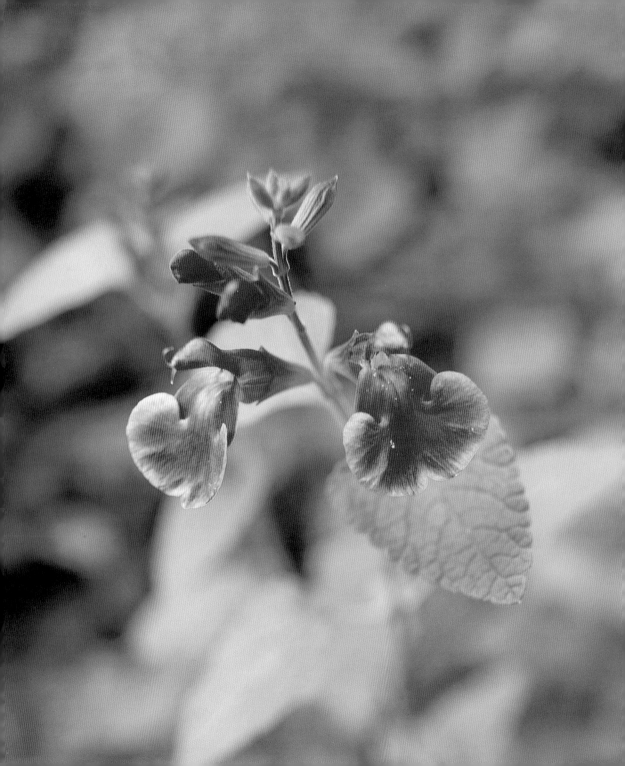

dry-country sages

inviting

Dry-country sages include some of the most desirable plants in the dryland gardener's palette. Autumn sage in particular is enjoying a vogue these days, with new forms appearing each season in plant catalogs and nurseries. Although most wild forms are red-flowered, gardeners have persistently selected and crossbred color breaks, expanding the range to include delicate, creamsicle oranges and peachy pastels. So far, only a few of these new named forms have found their way into the trade, but many small specialty nurseries list pink, peach, and pastel coral forms. The smaller mail-order nurseries don't generally have spiffy catalogs, but they are always the first to find and offer great new plants.

In chapter 1 you met the exciting group of natural hybrids between autumn sage (*S. greggii*) and littleleaf sage (*S. microphylla*), clustered as *S. x jamensis*. The Jame sages are just as inviting to gardeners as they are to bees, butterflies, and hummingbirds, and for good reason. Since the very recent discovery of several Jame sage populations in Mexico (during the late 1980s), this lively cross has displayed an ever-increasing variety of color forms. Delicate form, sturdy constitution, and astonishing color range won Jame sage instant acclaim. Barely a decade after its initial discovery, gardeners can find over a dozen named forms available, both from mail-order catalogs and small specialty nurseries. Like both parents, the Jame sages are highly drought tolerant once established.

Littleleaf sage is among the longest flowering of all sages, making it extremely popular with gardeners who want to attract wildlife. As with the Jame sages, littleleaf sages are highly attractive to both insects and hummingbirds. Not plants for small gardens, these bushy dryland sages become semiwoody in time and may develop into large (4- to

6-foot) shrubs in milder regions. 'Kew Red', perhaps the most widely grown form, can remain in bloom for seven or more months at a stretch, which is quite a feat for a plant that requires very little water to supply such abundance.

Gentian sage (*S. patens*) is not quite such a workhorse, but its prolific floral displays bring rare and most desirable shades of true blue to beds and borders. Common throughout much of Mexico, gentian sage is decidedly drought tolerant once established but grows better than either *S. greggii* or *S. microphylla* where winters are wet.

These handsome, hardworking plants will be embraced eagerly by gardeners wherever water use is restricted, whether by nature or by intelligent choice or even by law. At this point, relatively few gardeners need to face this issue, but within a few years this situation is likely to change. Indeed, in many parts of the country, it is already changing. As environmental laws develop and the human population continues to increase, more communities will face limitations on resources long considered to be infinite.

Water is of course a renewable resource, especially when we gardeners take on the careful stewardship of our property. Water from gardens that are not polluted with herbicides and pesticides replenishes groundwater without contamination. When we design gardens that require only minimal amounts of supplemental watering during high-use periods, we can make a significant contribution to preserving water quality and conserving this invaluable resource. The dry-country sages rank among the best choices we can make if we want to use water wisely.

Littleleaf Sage *Salvia microphylla* ZONES 8 | 9

In England, littleleaf sage is called Graham's sage and has been a popular border beauty for over a century. Plants from high-mountain regions tend to be more frost tolerant than those from lower altitudes, and hybrids vary in vigor and hardiness. Fine textured and small leaved, this mounding shrub is semievergreen in mild climates. The slim little leaves are a matte, silvery green and silky to the touch, releasing a brisk, pungent scent when handled and after a warm rain. To keep this sage tidy and compact, prune long branches back by half (or more) in late winter or early spring. The slim, tubular firecracker flowers are magenta red in the species, while the subspecies *S. m. neurepia* is more compact, with greener leaves and clear red flowers.

LITTLELEAF SAGE IN THE GARDEN This long-blooming plant grows best where winters are mild and summers are warm. In England and parts of the Pacific Northwest, littleleaf sage may reach 5 or 6 feet in height and girth if given a sheltered spot against a sunny wall. There it may bloom for six months (early summer through fall), producing wave after wave of hot red flowers that are often alive with hummingbirds. In open spots (and in hotter, drier California), it seldom exceeds half that size and tends to bloom in bursts rather than nonstop. In cooler climates, littleleaf sage may be grown as a container plant and brought indoors for the winter. Often grown as an annual, this willing worker blooms hard the first year and makes a rewarding bedding or container plant. As such, it appreciates border-beauty treatment, enjoying rich, well-drained soil amended with plenty of compost and a regular supply of summer water, but where hardy, littleleaf sage prefers less deluxe conditions, living longest though growing less densely and blooming less ardently in leaner, drier conditions.

PLEASING PARTNERSHIPS Littleleaf sage makes lovely, loose billows that contrast strikingly with architectural fans of spiky yuccas and low sprawls of sweet sumac, *Rhus aromatica*, whose flaming fall foliage sets off the sage's late blooms with flare. Underplant littleleaf sage with flowing sheets of low-growing blue Hebe 'Carl Teschner' and thick mats of creeping woolly thyme.

NAMED FORMS OF LITTLELEAF SAGE Named forms are widely available in England but harder to find in North America. Here are the most common:

ALBA
White flowers; compact

CERRO POTOSI
Singing, magenta-red flowers

MARASCHINO
Cherry red flowers; bushy

ROSITA
Bubble-gum pink flowers; shrubby

WILD WATERMELON
Hot pink flowers; shrubby

Autumn Sage *Salvia greggii* ZONES 6 | 7

With a wide native distribution from Texas into Mexico, it's not surprising that some forms of autumn sage are hardier than others. The species is also quite variable in size and shape, producing compact, foot-tall plants with red flowers, rangy 4-footers with white ones, and almost everything in between. The airy flower stalks bear their blooms at the tips from midsummer into autumn. Typical plants have small, fine-textured, glossy foliage of medium or grayish green. In the warmest areas, autumn sage is an evergreen or semideciduous shrub, while at the cooler edge of its range, it acts as a hardy perennial. Where it grows shrublike, trim back leggy stems in late spring to promote bushiness.

AUTUMN SAGE IN THE GARDEN Like littleleaf sage, autumn sage thrives in warm summers and mild winters. In cooler regions, winter protection of airy mulch and fir branches will help bring the plants through undamaged. Where summers are cool, autumn sage prefers an open, sunny spot, preferably one with reflected heat from sidewalks and patios. Autumn sage makes an adaptable container plant and may be sheltered in a garage or frost-free greenhouse over the winter. The many hybrids bloom generously enough to make them worthy annuals in very cold places. If grown as an annual, autumn sage prefers good, well-amended garden soil and regular water in dry periods. Periodic deadheading will increase the length and quantity of bloom. Where hardy, autumn sage does best in gritty, well-drained soil and becomes increasingly drought tolerant with age.

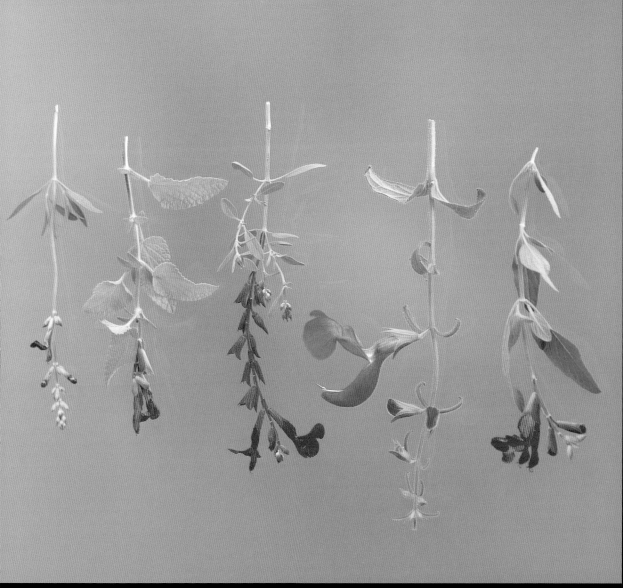

Sage *from left to right*

1 *Salvia greggii*
   NUEVO LEON

2 *Salvia microphylla*
   var. neurepia

3 *Salvia greggii*
   FURMAN'S RED

4 *Salvia patens*
   CAMBRIDGE BLUE

5 *Salvia microphylla*
   TWO TONE

Pleasing partnerships Long- and late-blooming autumn sages will mingle happily with rosy daylilies and purple coneflowers all summer, then bloom on to feed the foliar flames of fall. The blue, purple, pink, coral, and yellow forms all work beautifully with dusky-leaved perennials like *Eupatorium x* 'Chocolate' and murky *Aster lateriflorus* 'Prince', as well as smoke- and thundercloud-colored sedums like 'Vera Jameson' and 'Bertram Anderson'. Hot red versions look delicious with purple butterfly bushes, tall sheaves of big-belled *Crocosmia* 'Lucifer', and copper *Carex buchananii*.

Named forms of autumn sage Autumn sage is increasingly popular and new named forms appear each season. Here are a few of the best:

BRILLIANT ROSE
Rose-red flowers; shrubby (to 24 inches)

CORAL
Warm salmon-coral flowers; to 24 inches

FURMAN'S RED
Sizzling pinky-red flowers; to 24 inches

LIPSTICK
Gleaming red flowers; to 24 inches

PURPLE
Vivid violet-purple flowers; to 24 inches

PURPLE PASTEL
Soft, grayed-purple flowers, late bloomer; to 24 inches

CHIFFON
Buttery yellow flowers; to 30 inches

DESERT BLAZE
Hot red flowers, cream variegated foliage; to 24 inches

HOT PINK
Lively pink flowers, long bloomer; 2–3 feet

NUEVO LEON
Rich purple flowers with white throat blotch; to 30 inches

PURPLE HAZE
Smoky purple flowers, long bloomer; 2–3 feet

SAN TAKAO
Smoky soft-pink flowers; to 24 inches

Gentian Sage *Salvia patens* ZONE 8

Central Mexico is home to the sparkling blue *S. patens,* a tender perennial often grown as an annual. In mild parts of England and the maritime Northwest, garden forms of gentian sage may reach 3 or 4 feet in height and girth, particularly if given the shelter of a warm, south-facing wall. In hotter, drier places, plants may be 1 or 2 feet high and wide. The gray-green leaves are small and neatly arrayed up the slim stalks, which bear alternate pairs of blue flowers in sequence from midsummer into autumn. Gentian sage forms plump, tuberlike roots that may be lifted and stored like dahlias in fall where this charming plant is not hardy.

GENTIAN SAGE IN THE GARDEN Gentian sage makes a generous contribution to the flow of blue in bed and border. Its neat habit, the dazzling quality of its colors, and its generosity of bloom have made gentian sage a beloved border plant in England for well over a century. Where summers are cool (as in England, the Pacific Northwest, and maritime gardens), gentian sage takes full sun with pleasure. In areas of hot summers, the vivid blue flowers will cook if not protected by afternoon shade. Gentian sage prefers good garden soil, well amended with compost and aged dairy manure; regular summer water will keep flowers coming in steady progression all season long. Deep mulch and a light covering of fir boughs will help bring gentian sage through harsh winters. An occasional bit of pinching and deadheading keep it dapper all season.

PLEASING PARTNERSHIPS Gentian sage's clean, clear blues sing in the garden, especially when it is partnered with butter yellow *Coreopsis* 'Moonbeam' and sherbety yarrows (*Achillea*) such as 'Coronation Gold', 'Sandstone', and 'Orange Queen'. Clean white butterfly weed, *Asclepias* 'Ice Ballet', and shaggy white masterwort (*Astrantia major*) also keep company well with blue gentian sage, with taller sprays of lacy white goatsbeard (*Aruncus aethusifolius*) tucked behind them all. White or blue forms pair elegantly with fluffy silver mound (*Artemisia schmidtiana*) and spires of deep blue monkshood (*Aconitum*).

ALBA
White flowers; 2–4 feet

CAMBRIDGE BLUE
Soft, pale blue flowers; 2–4 feet

GUANAJUATO
Large, vivid blue flowers; 3–4 feet

WHITE TROPHY
Icy white flowers; 2–4 feet

A SAGE IS A SAGE IS... AN ARTEMISIA

White Sage *Artemisia ludoviciana* ZONE 5

When is a sage not a sage? When it is a member of the desert artemisias. Sacred to Artemis, goddess of the hunt, artemisias are members of the great composite clan, related to tarragon and mugworts. Most of the 300 or so artemisia species found around the world are pungently aromatic. Not surprisingly, artemisias have been associated with worship rituals in many cultures.

Smudging sages are native to the American Southwest, where they grow in profusion. The riders of the purple sage were galloping through billows of *Artemisia filifolia*, or Texan sand sage, whose thready foliage has a purple-blue cast at sunrise and sunset. Big sagebrush, *A. tridentata*, is a taller, pewter gray shrub that populates American deserts and dry prairies from lower Canada into Mexico. White sage, *A. ludoviciana* (also known as *A. purshiana*), is a lower-growing, silvery shrub with many garden forms, some of which are runaways in rich soil.

White sage is the most adaptable of the desert sages and is easily grown in almost any garden setting. The old standard, 'Silver King' is an infamous rowdy in good border soil, but invaluable in tough situations where dry, gravelly soil and full sun might daunt lesser plants. A newer form, 'Valerie Finnis' is elegantly silvery in color and lacy in form and more restrained in manner. This lovely garden plant can be used to scent potpourri and is prized for craft use in making dried wreaths and flower arrangements. The foliage can be used in ceremonial smudges for purification rituals.

Ceremonial Smudges

In North America, many western tribes of native people burned bundles of dried sage and cedar as a traditional way to cleanse a troubled environment. Today, many use sage "smudges" to symbolically purify a new home.

How to Gather and Dry Desert Sage

Harvest any aromatic desert sage in summer or early autumn, whether plants are in or out of flower. Cut pieces 10–12 inches long, choosing slim stems that are firm but flexible. Store in bags or loose bundles to keep foliage intact and use within in a day or two of gathering.

How to Make a Sage Smudge

Smudge bundles are made with fresh sage. For each smudge, bundle about a dozen sage pieces with a rubber band into a bunch about ½ inch in diameter (the bushy parts of the stems will be much wider). Weave the smudge with two multiple-strand pieces of embroidery floss about 6 feet long. To make this easier, wind the floss into small bundles and fasten with rubber bands.

Tie the silk strands together at one end, then make another small knot about 2 inches farther down their length, creating a small loop for hanging the sage bundles as they dry. Now tie the silk floss tightly around the sage stems, making a double knot. As the sage dries, it will shrink, so this first knot should be as tight as possible.

Wind the two strands of floss around the sage twigs, wrapping each in opposite directions. Wrap one strand 8–10 times, leave a ¼-inch gap, then wrap the other strand in a similar manner, or experiment with other patterns as you prefer. Work tightly so the sage stays put as it dries. Bundle the sage the whole way down the length of the stems, or leave the bottom part loose, which looks especially pretty when flowering stems are used. Hang smudges by their loops in a dry, airy place out of direct sunlight for a few weeks.

Smudging Ceremonies

Though the specifics of smudging rituals vary, the principles remain the same. To cleanse and purify a room and home, the smudger focuses intention on the space to be cleansed. The smudge is lit like incense; it catches alight, then the tiny flames die down, and the pungent, aromatic smoke is waved throughout the space.

Smudging with Salvias

Traditional North American smudges are made from artemisias, but European traditions use salvias. Smoke from the dried leaves of clary sage (*Salvia sclarea*) and common sage (*S. officinalis*) was considered powerfully cleansing. Smudges may be made with either or both of these sages and both smell quite pleasant when combined with cedar, as is common in several North American traditions.

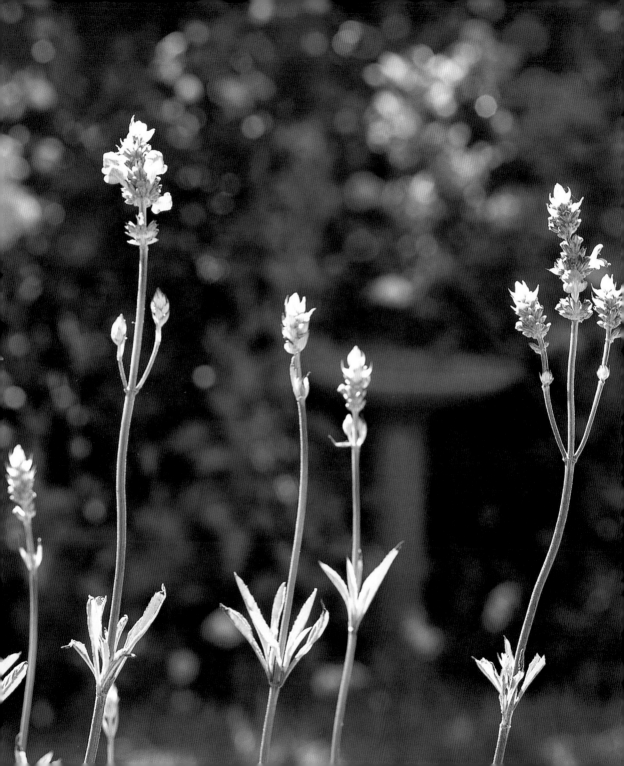

late-blooming sages

Big Blue Sage *Salvia guaranitica*

Bog Sage *S. uliginosa*

Indigo Spires Sage *S. 'Indigo Spires'*

robust

Most gardeners are familiar with the bedding and border salvias, willing workers that bloom all summer long. This extensive family also includes a number of reliable season extenders, sages that will carry the torch of color well into autumn. The big, bold sages profiled in this chapter bring sheaves of brilliant blue blossoms to the fall garden, matching the flames of fall foliage with their own intensity. These late starters are most effective where Indian summer is prolonged and dry, but even in the soggy maritime Northwest, they handily earn their place in the border.

Big blue sage (*S. guaranitica*) comes by its common name honestly. Happy plants can achieve the bulk and height of a good-sized maiden grass (*Miscanthus*), and indeed, the two plants make a potently handsome partnership. All forms have significant floral power, but the outsized, glowing flowers of 'Purple Majesty' carry across the garden with remarkable strength, as do the old-gold leaves of 'Omaha Gold' (named for its finder, not the city).

A haze of sky blue blossoms turn bog sage (*S. uliginosa*) into a gentle backdrop for deeper-toned asters and gilded grasses. Though they begin in midsummer, bog sage's flowers arrive in profusion just as summer's show is winding down. One of my favorite sights is a stand of bog sage in fall, long stems swaying under a burden of bees. The flowers are not strongly scented (though the leaves smell a bit minty), but they are endlessly attractive to hummingbirds as well as hosts of pollinating insects.

A chance hybrid, 'Indigo Spires' is the find of a lifetime for many gardeners. Compact and sturdy, the plants produce astonishingly large bloom stalks (some are nearly 2 feet long). Such length enables 'Indigo Spires' to bloom with abandon from midsummer well into autumn, looking fresh the whole time. Like all the sages in this chapter, 'Indigo Spires' is fast-growing but on the tender side. To be sure of keeping a steady supply of any or all of these choice plants, take plant divisions or root or rhizome cuttings in late summer.

To do this, gently loosen the soil around the base of the plants with a garden fork. The youngest growth (which makes the best divisions) will be at the outer edges of the plants. Expose the roots; then make clean cuts with a sharp garden knife, removing 2- to 3-inch chunks of rooted plant. Pot these up at once in well-drained potting soil. Water new divisions in well and place them out of direct light until they recover from transplant shock. As winter approaches, move them to a sheltered sunporch, a cold frame, or unheated greenhouse until spring.

The small rhizomes (fleshy storage roots) at the plant's skirts can be gently separated from the mother plant and potted up at the same depth as you found them in the soil. To keep the potting soil open-textured and well oxygenated, it is customary to use one part grit or coarse sand to two parts potting mix. Water new divisions in well and overwinter them as you would plant divisions. To take root cuttings from plants without rhizomes, slice off 2-inch chunks of thick, main root. Trim the bottom section (the bit farthest from the mother plant) at an angle to make a pointed tip. Pot root sections up in gritty soil, placing them with the slanted cut down (under the soil) and the flat cut (top) even with the soil level. Root cuttings are wintered over in the same manner as the others.

Big Blue Sage *Salvia guaranitica* ZONES 6 | 7

Native to South America, big blue sage has been grown in England and North America for well over a century. In the wild and in gardens, this handsome sage may stretch from 4 to 6 or even 8 feet depending on local conditions. Stiff, upright stems give big blue sage good form, but they are brittle and easily broken by wind in an exposed position. The fine-textured, tapered oval leaves are a fresh, deep green on top and somewhat hairy beneath, with a spicy, aniselike scent that is released at the slightest touch. The long stems bear quantities of large flowers in saturated shades of blue or purple, often set in dramatically dark calyces. Most forms bloom steadily from midsummer into fall.

BIG BLUE SAGE IN THE GARDEN One of the few sages that grows well in clay soils, big blue sage nonetheless grows best where drainage is good and will not tolerate standing water in winter. As an annual or perennial, it performs brilliantly in full sun and good garden soil, especially when watered through dry summers. Lean, sandy soils will require abundant amendment with compost and aged dairy manure to improve moisture retention for this plant. At the edge of its range, big blue sage is hardiest in warm summer regions with ample snow cover. To come through harsh winters, it requires perfect drainage and protection from frost heaves, such as a deep, airy mulch of shredded leaves and a loose covering of fir boughs. In cool regions, protect summer-rooted tip cuttings or autumn root divisions in a frost-free location over the winter. To take divisions, dig up pieces of the running roots, which have cylindrical nodules or storage rhizomes attached. Pot these up in fast-draining soil and protect from frost.

PLEASING PARTNERSHIPS Big blue sage flowers are an intense color that glows magically in subtle settings. The old-gold lace of golden cutleaf elder (*Sambucus racemosa* 'Plumosa Aurea') sets off the bright flowers beautifully, as will sheaves of golden rain grass, *Stipa gigantea*, and tall stands of willow-leaved butter daisy, *Bidens heterophylla.* The jewel blues also mingle deliciously with silky late-blooming Japanese anemones in rose or white and clouds of smoky *Aster novae-angliae* 'Purple Dome'. Underplant big blue sage with billows of dusky *Euphorbia dulcis* 'Chameleon' and running spills of *Geranium wallichianum* 'Buxton's Variety'.

ARGENTINA SKIES
Hazy, soft-blue flowers, starts early; 4–6 feet

BLUE ENIGMA
Ocean blue flowers, green calyces,
starts early; 4–6 feet

BLACK AND BLUE
Cobalt flowers, black calyces,
late starter; 3–4 feet

OMAHA GOLD
Old-gold leaf margins, cobalt flowers,
black calyces; 3–6 feet

PURPLE MAJESTY
Tender hybrid, large purple flowers,
late starter; 4–6 feet

Bog Sage *Salvia uliginosa* ZONES 7 | 8

Introduced at the same time as big blue sage, this South American beauty took a century to gain a following and still lacks named forms. In warm, sheltered gardens, this upright, graceful plant may reach 6 or 8 feet in height and the long, supple stems sway with the elegance of bamboo on any breeze. Each is clothed in slim, willowlike leaves that are faintly hairy below and vivid green above. The airy but abundant flowers are set on short bloom stalks nestled into stubby green calyces. The blossoms are pale blue and white, their wide lips penciled with white whiskers. They appear in bountiful bursts from mid-summer until frost and may continue through winter in very mild years.

BOG SAGE IN THE GARDEN Despite the common name, bog sage will not tolerate standing water in winter, but grows with alacrity in soils that remain uniformly moist in summer. Where hardy, its rapid growth can be slowed by giving it a drier spot in well-drained soil, where it will appreciate receiving supplemental water in dry summers. Bog sage is an adaptable plant that takes a wide range of conditions in stride, though it blooms most abundantly when given full sun and well-drained soil amended with compost and mulched with shredded leaves. Where it seems to vanish in winter, try baiting early in spring with Sluggo to protect the young shoots, which can be ravaged by hungry slugs and snails. In cool regions, summer-rooted tip cuttings or autumn divisions of the spreading root rhizomes may be overwintered in a frost-free greenhouse or garage.

PLEASING PARTNERSHIPS Delicate blue-and-white bog sage looks smashing with tall white Japanese anemones and a calico aster, 'Lady in Black', whose dark leaves and dusty pink flowers make the soft blues sparkle. For more drama, pair it with *Cimicifuga* 'Black Negligee', a lacy bugbane whose white flowers are sumptuously scented in fall.

Indigo Spires Sage *Salvia 'Indigo Spires'* ZONE 9

'Indigo Spires' arose as a spontaneous hybrid at California's Huntington Botanical Gardens. Where hardy, it makes a bushy, mounding shrub 3–5 feet tall and wide, its relaxed arms heavy with bloom. Small but profuse purple-blue flowers are set in violet calyces, and the same rich purple infuses the leaf veins and stems. The glossy green leaves are long, tapering ovals, lightly scalloped at the edges and delicately furred below. When brushed, they release a pungent, wild scent that is also noticeable after a warm rain.

Informal in habit, 'Indigo Spires' benefits from the support of stakes or plant hoops. Whether grown as a hardy shrub, a perennial, or as an annual, it blooms from early summer through fall. In the two decades since its introduction, 'Indigo Spires' has swept the country and hopped the ocean and is already considered a classic border plant.

INDIGO SPIRES SAGE IN THE GARDEN Like many quick growers, 'Indigo Spires' flourishes in full sun and generously amended soils that drain well. For best performance, water regularly during dry spells and apply half-strength fertilizer at least monthly from spring into midsummer. Pinching back the longest stems in late spring and early summer promotes bushiness, while frequent deadheading encourages continual bloom. Where hardy, trim stems back to a low framework in spring. Cuttings rooted in late summer or fall may be overwintered in a frost-free greenhouse.

PLEASING PARTNERSHIPS The saturated purple-blue flowers of 'Indigo Spires' set off warm yellows and golds to perfection. For a long season of contrast, interplant several with the sturdy border shrub, *Spirea* 'Goldflame', adding some copper and burnt orange Peruvian lily, *Alstroemeria* 'Yvonne', in front. To play up the blue theme, partner 'Indigo Spires' with the soft blue monkshood, *Aconitum* 'Stainless Steel', blue globe thistles such as *Echinops* 'Veitch's Blue', and blue magellan grass (*Elymus magellanicus*).

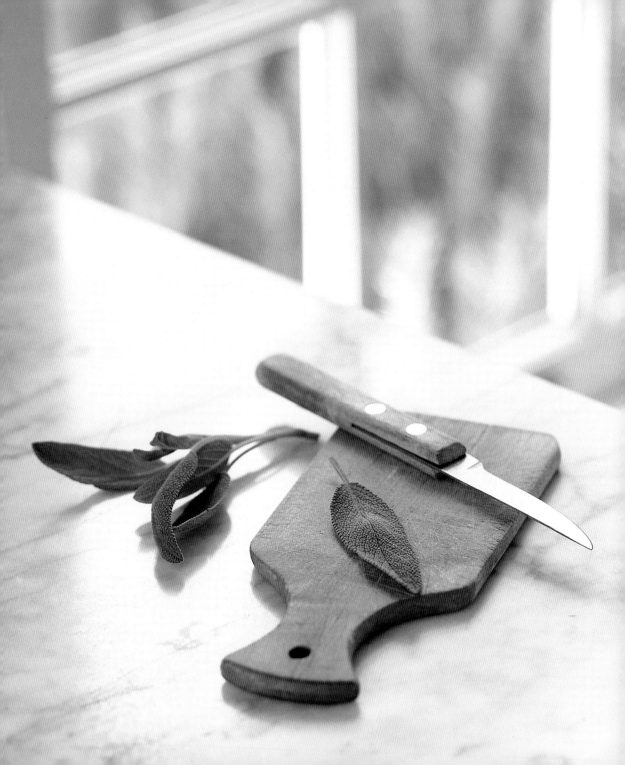

4

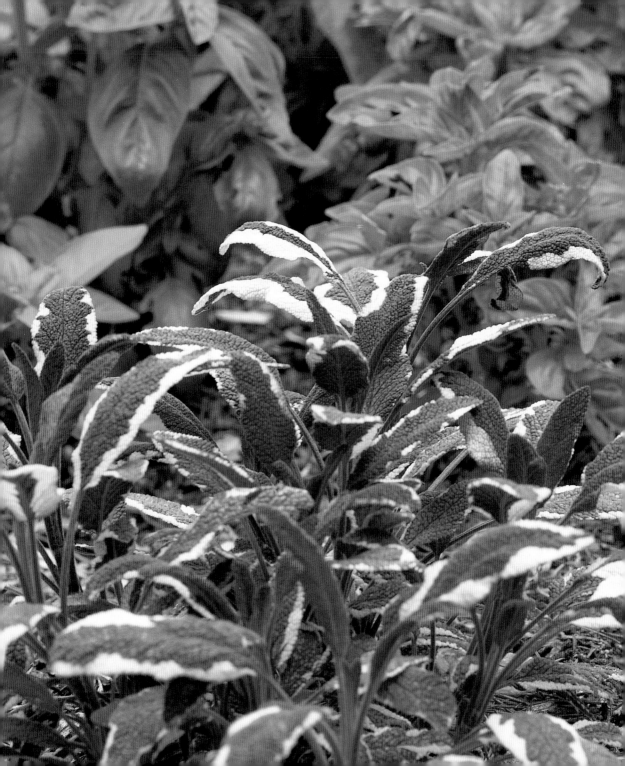

culinary sages

Common Sage *Salvia officinalis*

Fruit Sage *S. dorisiana*

Pineapple Sage *S. elegans 'Scarlet Pineapple' (syn. S. rutilans)*

savory

Flowering sages may take pride of place in ornamental beds and borders, but certain of the culinary sages are at least as popular as the bountiful bloomers. For hundreds of years, scented salvia foliage has been a treasured ingredient in countless home recipes around the world. In countries with climates and cultures as diverse as those of England and Guatemala, salvias have long-standing traditions for both culinary and medicinal use as well as their ornamental role.

Of all the hundreds of salvia species, the three profiled in this chapter are outstanding for their savory, scented foliage. All remain in continuous, daily use in their native lands. All have also made their way around the world to be enjoyed by gardeners and cooks in other climes.

Many authorities assert that common sage (*S. officinalis*) was introduced in England by Roman invaders. The use of sage is well documented through the Dark Ages, and early garden books, such as *Gerard's Herbal,* offer as many medicinal applications for sage leaves and blossoms as culinary ones. Common sage came to the New World with the first settlers and has never since fallen from favor. While most salvia species produce relatively few variant forms, this is one of the mutable sages. Colorful, tasty forms abound, some, like 'Purpurascens', of ancient heritage, others, like 'Berggarten', of quite modern introduction.

Honduran fruit sage (*S. dorisiana*) is a relative newcomer, having only been introduced to European gardeners in 1950. In half a century, the fruity, flavorful foliage has traveled from bed and border to the kitchen and the bath. In England, Europe, and North America, fruit sage has become a common ingredient in all sorts of concoctions, from teas and sorbets to hand creams and bath salts. Dried foliage is often found in potpourris and gives herbal bath blends a gentle, fruity scent.

Pineapple sage, *S. elegans* 'Scarlet Pineapple' (known for over a century as *S. rutilans*), has been prized since the late 1800s for its sumptuously pineapple-scented foliage, which Victorians used to perfume fingerbowls and to flavor fruit salads. A few leaves of pineapple sage will add a mellowing sweetness to summery iced teas, whether black, green, or herbal. In its native home (Mexico and Guatemala), pineapple sage leaves are sometimes chewed to sweeten the breath.

You will learn more about growing and uses for these "sages of service" both below and in chapter 6, where you will find many recipes to try out. As you will see, all of these useful plants have multiple uses in cookery, herbal treatments, aromatherapy, and crafts. Try a few of the recipes for yourself, and you will understand precisely how these willing workers earn their way into gardens everywhere.

All three are considered to be "crossover" plants, so you can make them as welcome in your ornamental borders as in your kitchen garden beds. Like the previous chapters, this one includes cultural information and partnership ideas, but here you will also learn how to gather, dry, and store these serviceable sages for culinary and other uses.

Common Sage *Salvia officinalis* ZONE 5

Common (or Garden) sage has been cultivated for several millennia, especially where it occurs naturally (throughout Europe, from Spain to the Balkan peninsula and into Asia Minor). Historically, sage was valued as a healing herb with many virtues and was widely used to treat respiratory and digestive ailments. Women treasured sage for regulating menstrual difficulties, men valued it to increase virility, and everyone used it to heal sore throats or swollen gums.

The specific epithet *officinalis* is common among herbs as it was traditionally used to indicate plants sold for medicinal purposes. Also a popular home remedy, sage foliage was eaten by mothers-to-be to ensure a healthy pregnancy and successful childbirth, while sage teas were recommended for strengthening the memory, clarifying the mind, and cleansing a stuffy head. Sage mouthwash not only sweetened the breath and helped heal canker sores but also imparted wisdom to one's words. Sage tea was also held to be a spring tonic to cleanse the blood and a common treatment for bothersome head colds.

One of several herbs held sacred to Athena, goddess of wisdom, sage was widely grown in Greece and throughout the Mediterranean basin. Sage leaves were burned at alters when prayers were made for guidance and wisdom. Ancient Romans ate fresh sage to increase wisdom, preserve health, and live longer lives, and old folks drank sage tea to strengthen body, mind, and memory. A famous Roman proverb held that the gardener who grew sage would never die. Sage was also used in the brewing of special beers to promote masculine health. In England and France, sage beers were the preferred drink of farmers and fieldworkers for several centuries and were considered to be especially health-building during the winter months. In both countries, fresh sage foliage was frequently used to flavor the plain bread and cheese that made up much of the daily diet of the lower classes.

Common sage is a traditional cooking herb, most often used to flavor roasted pork and poultry. Small amounts of fresh or dried sage also add savor to soups, stews, dishes using dry beans, and vegetable stir-fries.

COMMON SAGE IN THE GARDEN A low-growing, spreading shrub, common sage seldom exceeds 2 feet in height but may reach 3 to 5 feet in girth over time. The stems are woolly with gray or white hairs, and the foliage may be green or gray, purple or golden, or attractively variegated. The flowers are also variable, and though blue is most common, seedlings may bloom purple, pink, or white.

This indispensable herb is hardiest and best looking when grown in full sun and lean, well-drained soils. Where native soils are heavy (clay based), common sage thrives in raised beds of fast-draining gritty soil. Sage grows well in coastal and windswept gardens, especially in light or sandy soils. In rich border soils, sage may deteriorate quickly, lasting only three or four years. Even in good conditions, common sage generally has an effective border life of five to six years. After that, the shrubs tend to grow lank and leggy. To keep them compact, trim stems in midsummer when you harvest the foliage. However, do not cut back into old wood (bare stems), for they will not resprout. Always leave at least an inch or two of lower stem with its leaves intact.

Where winters are cold, common sage may be grown in large containers, such as half barrels, and stored in a garage or sun porch during the winter months. Though most forms of common sage are hardy to zone 5, the weaker, slow-growing variegated forms may die out in persistently wet winters or when sudden cold snaps occur after a mild autumn. The hardiest forms include 'Berggarten', 'Herrenhausen', and 'Holt's Mammoth'.

NAMED FORMS OF COMMON SAGE

ALBIFLORA
Slim foliage, white flowers

AUREA
Soft golden foliage, blue flowers, slow grower

BERGGARTEN
Bold gray foliage, strong grower, excellent border plant, very long lived (8–10 years)

COMPACTA
Dwarf plant (about 8 inches); narrow gray-green foliage

CRISPA
Creamy variegated leaves with curly margins

GRETE STOLZE
Slim, tapered, silvery foliage; mauve flowers

HERRENHAUSEN
Large gray leaves, dense habit, good border plant

HOLT'S MAMMOTH
Broad gray leaves, compact, good border plant

ICTERINA
Chartreuse foliage with old-gold margins, slow grower

KEW GOLD
Dainty, pale-yellow and chartreuse foliage, fair grower; may revert to 'Icterina'; compact (to 12 inches)

LATIFOLIA
Narrow gray leaves, blue flowers

MILLERI
Mottled and splotched burgundy foliage, slow grower

PURPURASCENS
Frosted purple leaves, excellent garden plant

PURPURASCENS VARIEGATA
Cream-splashed sport of 'Purpurascens'

ROBIN HILL
Cream-marbled red-purple leaves; compact

RUBRIFLORA
Narrow, strappy gray-green foliage, red flowers

SALICIFOLIA
Long, slender gray foliage, fine-textured border plant

STURNINA
Green-and-white foliage

TENUIOR
Ribbony gray leaves

TRICOLOR
Leaves gray-green, cream to butter, and rose

HARVESTING COMMON SAGE Common sage can be harvested all year round for fresh use where the shrub is hardy. Sage foliage should be gathered in the morning of a dry, sunny day, preferably at least two or three days after the last rainstorm, to ensure that the leaves are properly dry and not waterlogged. If leaves are to be dried, avoid the oldest and youngest leaves, selecting mature, unblemished foliage of medium size. Gather foliage for drying before the flowers are fully formed. To maintain the health of an evergreen plant, don't remove more than about 25 percent of the total foliage. Where summers are long and autumns mild, you may harvest two crops of foliage (in early summer and early autumn, when sage may rebloom) without harming the plant. Where winters are harsh and summers short, a single harvest in midsummer will be less stressful to the plant.

Mature foliage contains more essential oils than old or immature foliage, which does not dry as well as fully developed leaves. Once plants have bloomed, the level of essential oils (and thus the fullest flavor) diminishes somewhat. However, fresh leaves of common sage may be used at any time for flavoring soups, stews, and stuffings.

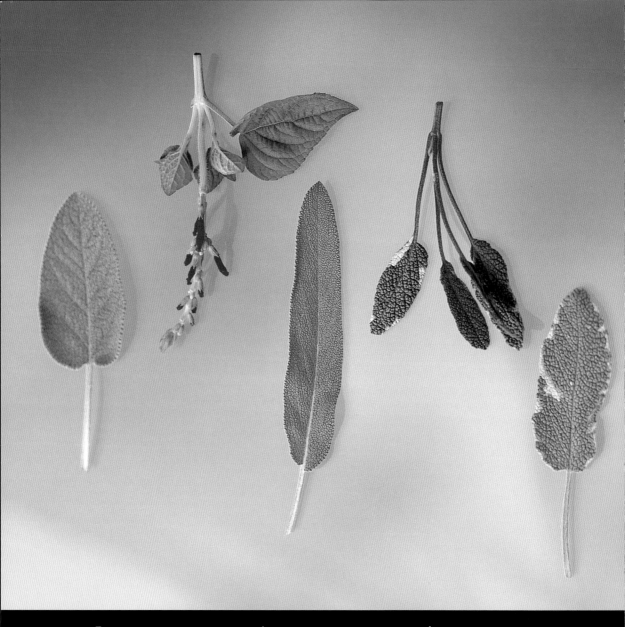

Sage *from left to right*

1 *Salvia officinalis 'Berggarten'*
BERGGARTEN

2 *Salvia elegans*
PINEAPPLE SAGE

3 *Salvia officinalis*
COMMON SAGE

4 *Salvia officinalis 'Tricolor'*
TRICOLOR

5 *Salvia officinalis 'Aurea'*
GOLDEN SAGE

If you are pruning your plants to keep them compact, shear the outer portion of each stem, taking care not to cut back into old wood (bare stems). Strip the leaves off the stems before drying. Old and discolored foliage should be added to the compost heap. Young, tender, and undersized leaves can be used fresh in salads, teas, and stir-fries but will not dry as well as mature foliage.

DRYING AND STORING COMMON SAGE Dry a single layer of sage leaves on racks (the wire cooling racks for baked goods work very well) with a layer of clean newspaper underneath to catch any foliage that falls through the wire. Dry the leaves in a cool, dark room, or at least out of direct sunlight. It may take a week or more for the leaves to dry completely. When dry, sage leaves feel crisp and break cleanly when crumbled.

Dried sage may be stored in plain or dark glass jars with tightly closing lids, in cloth or paper bags, or in plastic bags. Dried foliage will keep well for several months if stored in a dark cupboard out of direct sunlight. For later use, dry foliage may be wrapped in a paper bag, then put in a sealed plastic zip-close bag and frozen for up to 6 months.

PLEASING PARTNERSHIPS Common sage looks attractive enough to be placed in ornamental borders as well as kitchen gardens. Purple sage (*'Purpurascens'*) ranks among the most attractive border plants in the garden, combining well with tall sedums such as 'Autumn Joy' and compact, silky ponytail grass, *Stipa tenuissima* (zone 6). Purple sage also makes a dramatic partner for ice blue Magellan grass, *Elymus magellanicus* (zone 5), a non-running lyme grass that deserves a front-line border position. Silvery gray 'Berggarten' sage makes a smooth, mounding shape that contrasts excitingly with swirls of coppery grasses like *Carex comans* 'Bronze' (zone 7) or sculptural spikes of hardy yucca. If your garden palette runs to pretty pastels, try pairing a rose-and-cream 'Tricolor' sage with a foam of pink, low-growing polyantha roses such as 'The Fairy' (zone 4).

Fruit Sage *Salvia dorisiana* ZONES 8 | 9

Native to the Honduras, this tender perennial is chiefly grown as an annual. Where winters are mild, fruit sage may act like a perennial, dying back to the root and reappearing with spring. In frost-free climates, it becomes shrublike, remaining evergreen and often flowering through the winter months. Dense and bushy, the multistemmed plants reach

3–4 feet in height, with long, oval leaves that feel thin and papery to the touch. The whole plant is slightly hairy and every part gives off the delightful fruity scent that reminds some noses of grapefruit and others of peaches. In late summer and autumn, the stem tips are covered with slim, tubular hot pink flowers that are magnets for hummingbirds and native solitary bees.

A fast grower in rich, well-drained soils, fruit sage appreciates afternoon shade where summers are hot but does best in full sun in cool, coastal gardens. Mulch helps keep fruit sage growing happily where early summer nights are cool and also keeps the roots moister during the heat of high summer. When fruit sage is grown in containers, offer regular feedings of half-strength fertilizer and winter over indoors.

PLEASING PARTNERSHIPS   Boldly built fruit sage stands up to dramatic partners like *Crocosmia* 'Lucifer' (zone 6) and the black-leaved dahlia, 'Bishop of Llandalf'. Echo its showy chartreuse bracts with lime-colored 'Sunfast' coleus and spills of *Helichrysum petiolare* 'Limelight'. Tone down its magenta blossoms with silvery *Artemisia ludoviciana* 'Valerie Finnis' (zone 5) and taller roseleaf sage, *Salvia involucrata* 'Bethellii' (see chapter 3).

HOW TO GATHER FRUIT SAGE   If you live where winters are frost free and fruit sage is an evergreen, harvest with discretion, removing no more than 25 percent of the whole plant and taking only mature leaves rather than old or younger ones. Where fruit sage is grown as an annual, reap the entire plant as summer wanes, drying the flowers for mixing in potpourri or dried tea blends and the foliage for use in teas, sachets, and bath salts. It's best to harvest foliage early in the morning of a dry, sunny day, preferably after a stretch of several dry, warm days.

DRYING AND STORING FRUIT SAGE   Dry the leaves and flowers in a single layer on drying racks placed over clean newspaper. Dry them out of direct sunlight, preferably in a cool, dark room. It may take two weeks for the leaves to dry completely. When dry, fruit sage leaves feel crisp and break cleanly when crumbled.

Store dried fruit sage in plain or dark glass jars with tightly closing lids. Dried foliage keeps well for several months if stored out of direct sunlight. Dry foliage may be wrapped in a paper bag, then put in a sealed plastic zip-close bag and frozen for up to six months.

Pineapple Sage *Salvia elegans 'Scarlet Pineapple'* ZONE 10

Grown as an annual, this tender perennial offers savory pineapple scent and flavor. Fans of fragrant foliage love to handle the fuzzy leaves, releasing wafts of refreshing, delicious scent. For over a century, this large-flowered, compact form of *Salvia elegans* has been called *Salvia rutilans*. Recently, botanists have shifted it back to the *S. elegans* family, even though it looks very different from the typical species plant. Its tropical origins make it most at home where summers are warm.

In its native home, pineapple sage is found at the edge of woodlands. In open settings, it appreciates some shade from hot sun. However, in cool, cloudy coastal gardens, it does best in full sun. Give it rich, well-drained soil amply amended with compost. Drought tolerant once established, young plants appreciate regular watering. Where hardy, pineapple sage may exceed 5 or 6 feet and makes a substantial evergreen shrub. A late bloomer, its red flowers are seldom seen where winter arrives early. Where autumn is protracted and mild, it draws hummingbirds to the garden until the first frost.

A selected form, *S.e.* 'Honey Melon', looks and smells distinctly different from the parent species. This compact dwarf (to 2 feet) has modestly running ways, particularly in warmer climates. It prefers good, well-drained garden soil with a warming blanket of compost mulch. Like pineapple sage, honey melon sage blooms from late summer into fall, often continuing on into winter where winters are mild. The small, fine-textured foliage has an enticingly sweet, fruity scent and tastes a bit more flavorful and somewhat sweeter than pineapple sage. This lovely tea herb makes a delicious addition to fruit salad and to light curries. The dried foliage can be added to potpourri or tea blends.

PLEASING PARTNERSHIPS Like all plants with fragrant foliage, pineapple sage is best used where passersby will brush against it. Tall and stately, this handsome herb consorts beautifully with arching maiden grass (*Miscanthus sinensis,* zone 4) and fountains of periwinkle blue *Aster frikartii* (zone 4). Place pineapple sage near a patio or seating area to attract hummingbirds. To create a dazzling summery perfume, underplant pineapple sage with mignonette and honey-scented sweet alyssum.

HOW TO GATHER, DRY, AND STORE PINEAPPLE SAGE

See Fruit Sage (page 79).

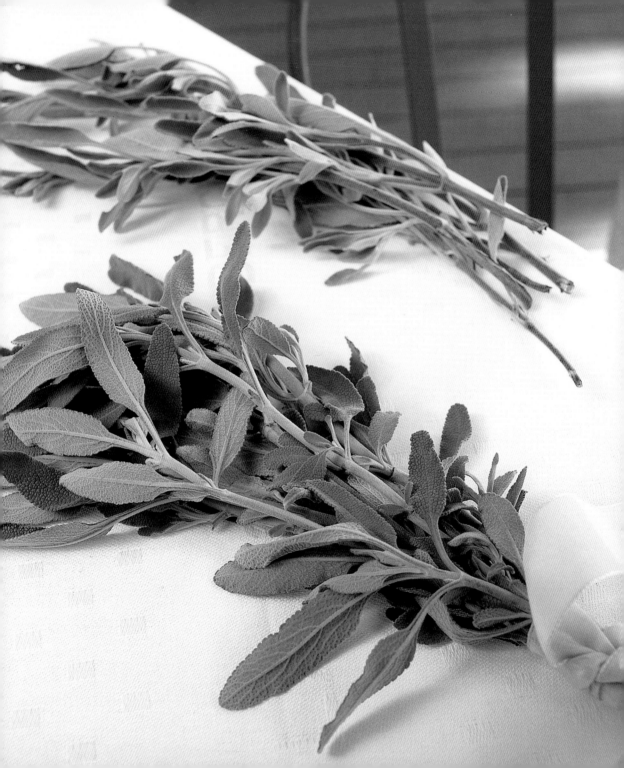

5

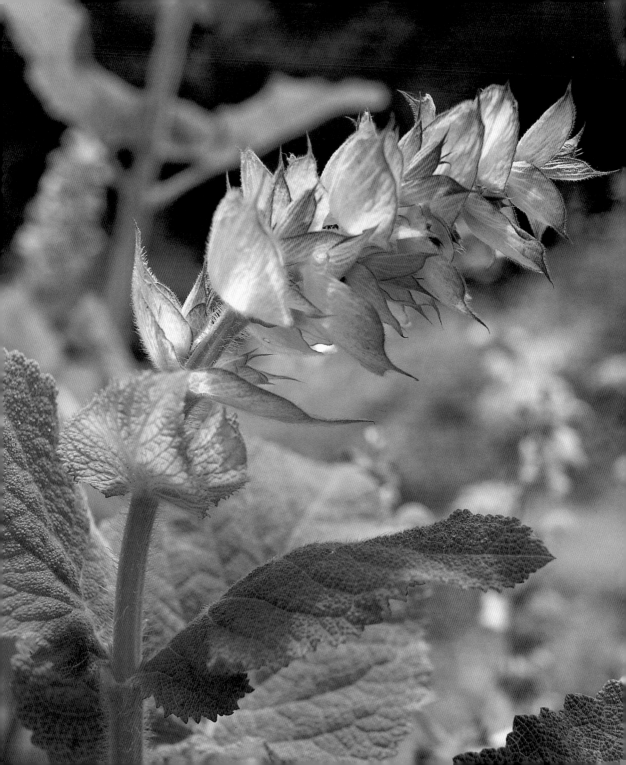

scented sages

Clary Sage *Salvia sclarea*

Cleveland Sage *S. clevelandii*

Spanish Sage *S. lavandulifolia*

aromatic

Many sages, ornamental and culinary, have fragrant foliage, but the three profiled in this chapter are outstanding in this respect. As usual in this handsome family, all are also gardenworthy in their own right. Any or all could be used in ornamental situations, particularly if you have a dry, sunny area where the soil is not particularly rich. Such a spot will suit these lean growers to the ground.

Indeed, all do best without much supplemental water and will grow best outside of any automatic sprinkler zones. None require fertilizing, other than a light annual mulching with an inch or so of compost or aged manure. All grow better in lean, gravelly, and well-drained soils than in generously amended borders. When life is too good for these plants, they grow lax and lanky instead of compact and densely furnished with foliage.

Their foliage will be most redolent when they are grown in full sun, preferably with a southern or western exposure. This matters most if you are growing the leaves for use in potpourri or to scent lotions and soaps, since the more sun you can give the plants, the more aromatic your product will be. If you just want to savor the scents in daily life, you'll find that any of these sages will accept less than ideal growing conditions.

If your garden doesn't present perfect spots for these sun lovers, look around the yard to find the warmest microclimate the property offers. Often the open, dry places along driveways, sidewalks, patios, or swimming pools receive a great deal of reflected light. In such a situation, your sage plants may enjoy significantly higher amounts of accumulated heat than in your garden beds.

Clary sage is the most adaptable of the bunch and will often grow happily even in the maritime Northwest (where "full sun" is an interesting concept).

Clary sage is also more tolerant of ordinary garden soil and seasonal damp than the others, both of which are decidedly unhappy where winters are long and persistently wet. Of these three scented sages, only clary sage has a lengthy heritage as a culinary and medicinal herb. Clary sage has been grown throughout Europe for centuries and came to North America with the Pilgrims, who used it to treat a number of common ailments.

Thanks to the enticing fragrance of their foliage, all three of these salvia species have historically been used for incense and purification ceremonies. Since the Dark Ages, clary sage has been considered to be a purifying herbal smudge herb (see chapter 5, 6, or sidebar on page 63). Both the dried foliage and the essential oil have a long history of use in religious ceremonies as well.

Cleveland sage, native to California, has been best known on the West Coast until recent years. As fragrance gardens have become increasingly popular, gardeners across the country and even across the water in England and Europe are learning to prize the fruity, pungent aroma of this natural beauty. It grows best in regions with a Mediterranean climate pattern of dry summers and wet winters and tends to suffer from root rot in warm, humid climates, especially where night temperatures remain high.

Spanish sage is more common in Europe than in North America but can be found at many nurseries that specialize in traditional medicinal herbs. This beautifully textured, silvery plant has lovely, dapper leaves that lend their piquant natural perfume to colognes and soaps, salves, and lotions of many kinds.

Clary Sage *Salvia sclarea* ZONE 5

Clary sage is frequent along roadsides and in meadows from southern Europe into central Asia. The common name is a corruption of "clear eye," a reference to a method for removing foreign objects from the eye that was traditional in ancient Greece as well as throughout Europe. A seed of clary sage was placed in the affected eye, causing the formation of a viscous fluid that captured the scratchy object so it could be removed painlessly along with the seed. Clary sage came to have many other uses, both high and lowly. Vatican sage was the old name for a highly aromatic form of clary sage used in incense for church services for over a thousand years. Beer made with clary sage instead of hops was potent enough to serve as an anesthetic when setting bones, because the patient would feel no pain (until later, presumably). Clary sage makes an enticingly aromatic wine vinegar with rich, Muscadet overtones. Do not, however, leave any foliage in the vinegar bottle to mellow, or the flavor will become unpleasantly strong. My favorite way to enjoy clary sage is as fritters. Crisp and delicious, these savory tidbits were held to be particularly healthful for those suffering from digestive complaints. These days, few of us consider fried food to be a particularly good cure for an upset stomach, but serve these snacks at a party and they will fly off the plate.

CLARY SAGE IN THE GARDEN Clary sage is a lusty grower, happiest with a lean, well-drained soil, full sun, and little or no supplemental water in summer. Though technically a perennial, clary sage acts as a self-sowing biennial in many gardens. Robust in height and vigor, it reaches 4 feet in height where pleased. Its multibranched arms hold dozens of flower spikes that rise, candelabra-like, above large, coarse basal foliage that continues partway up the square stems. The vivid green, deeply embossed leaves are gray green on the hairy underside and are the most fragrant part of the plant, though the flowers also offer scent and savor. The scent of both is aromatic rather than floral, and though generally pleasing, this potent perfume affects some noses unpleasantly, especially when the flowers are cut for the house. A batch of seedlings will bloom in a gentle, tweedy blend of white, pink, lavender, and blue, with showy, colored bracts that outlast the blossoms. If deadheaded regularly, clary sage blooms from early summer into fall. If left to flower unchecked, it blooms most heavily in early summer, then repeats quite reliably in autumn.

Clary sage in any form requires a fair amount of space, since the base foliage can be 3 or 4 feet across. The marvelously architectural Turkish sage, *Salvia sclarea 'Turkestanica'*, develops an even wider skirted rosette, so allow young plants plenty of elbow room in the border. This white-flowered Turkish sage has pale pink bracts, though a selected form, 'Alba', is clean white throughout. Turkish sage is even less perennial than clary and is most often sold as a biennial. To keep a steady supply coming, plant out youngsters two years running. Turkish sage will reseed somewhat, though it is less generous than clary sage. Seedlings of both are gobbled up by slugs, so it's wise to gather seed in fall and sow it in pots in spring to ensure a fresh supply of plants. You can protect young plants with a sprinkle of Sluggo, an ecologically safe slug bait based on coconut and iron phosphate that gives slugs anorexia without harming birds or pets.

PLEASING PARTNERSHIPS Soft-colored forms of clary sage make a bold front for tall bloomers such as Joe Pye weed (*Eupatorium fistulosum* 'Gateway') or queen of the prairie (*Filipendula rubra*). They also contrast well with purple coneflower (*Echinacea purpurea*) and low-growing pink roses such as 'Simplicity' or 'Bonica'. Turkish sage looks dramatic with bold-textured plants such as shrubby purple sand cherry (*Prunus x cistena* 'Purpurea') and the taller maiden grasses (*Miscanthus sinensis*). To make the most of its autumnal reprise, match Turkish sage with cascades of periwinkle blue frikart aster (*Aster x frikartii*) and airy towers of thousand aster plant, *Boltonia asteroides*, which comes in billowy white- or pink-flowered forms.

GATHERING AND DRYING CLARY SAGE Perennial clary sage can be gathered as generously as any annual herb for dried use. When used fresh, foliage should be picked as needed. Gather and dry clary sage as you would fruit sage (see chapter 4).

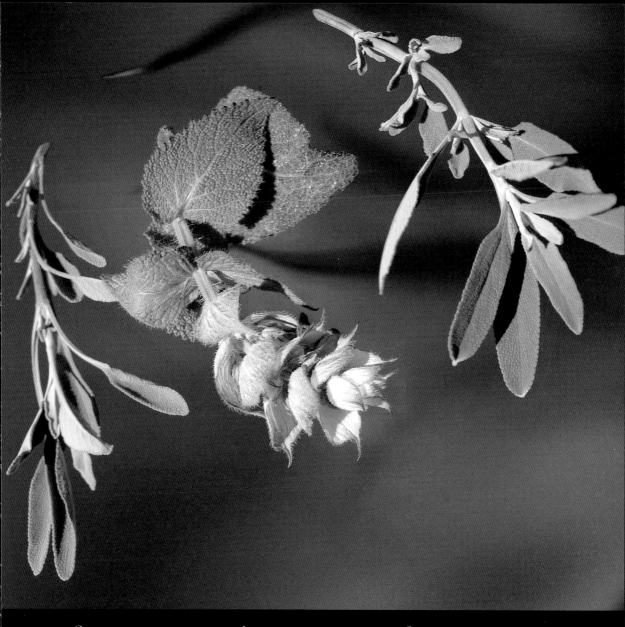

Sage *from left to right*

1 *Salvia apiana*
BEE'S BLISS

2 *Salvia sclarea*
CLARY SAGE

3 *Salvia clevelandii 'Aromas'*
CLEVELAND SAGE

Cleveland Sage *Salvia clevelandii* ZONE 8

Native from southern California into Baja California, Cleveland sage is a dramatically silvery shrub with rosy purple or bright blue flowers. The small, tapered oval foliage has a musky, cherry tobacco–like fragrance that is released freely in the air. When handled, the foliage gives off a stronger, deeper perfume with floral overtones. The leaves hold their scent well when dried, making them splendid ingredients in potpourri. In gardens where fragrant foliage is a specialty, Cleveland sage handily earns its spot, even if it must be grown as an annual. If container-grown plants are to be overwintered indoors, give them the most sunny windowsill available. Because overwatered plants will rot, provide quick-draining, well-aerated soil and water sparingly, only when soil is dry to the depth of an inch. Your reward will be a hauntingly aromatic fragrance that subtly permeates the room.

CLEVELAND SAGE IN THE GARDEN Cleveland sage thrives in lean soil and fast drainage, and it requires full sun and a good flow of air. It does well in windy sites and grows especially well in coastal gardens. In its native California, Cleveland sage forms a handsome and compact mound that ranges from 3 to 5 feet in height and girth. In milder climates, notably sheltered coastal gardens in northern California and southern Oregon, this silvery shrub may exceed 8 feet in height and 6 in width. In cooler climes where winters are wet and summers less hot (such as the Puget Sound area of Washington), Cleveland sage may grow a mere 1 to 2 feet high and wide, depending on the amount of summer heat it receives. Where winters are wet, Cleveland sage does best in raised beds with plenty of added grit. Where winter cold is severe, Cleveland sage must be grown as a container plant and overwintered indoors or in a well-ventilated greenhouse. High humidity does not agree with this native of the dry chaparral, though it enjoys hot summers and does not mind hot nights.

PLEASING PARTNERSHIPS Where Cleveland sage grows happily, it partners beautifully with evergreen Mediterranean herbs such as rosemary and lavender as well as spiky yuccas and agaves. Its silvery coloration contrasts potently with purple-leaved hebes and bronze or burgundy forms of New Zealand flax (*Phormium tenax*). In cooler climates, this well-mannered shrub combines attractively with architectural sea hollies and shapely grasses such as golden needle grass (*Stipa gigantea*), and zebra maiden grass (*Miscanthus sinensis* 'Stricta'). Grown as a container plant, Cleveland sage can be set, pot and all, into the border to cover gaps left by early bulbs that retreat into dormancy by summer. Set a trio of 1-by-1-inch sticks beneath the container to keep the dormant bulbs from rotting.

NAMED FORMS OF CLEVELAND SAGE

AROMAS
Medium blue, very fragrant foliage

SALVIA X 'BEE'S BLISS'
Hybrid with *S. leucophylla*, pinky lavender flowers

BETSY CLEBSCH
Pale to warm blue flowers, good form

POZO BLUE
Sparkling, bright blue flowers

SANTA CRUZ DARK
Deep, rich blue flowers

GATHERING AND DRYING CLEVELAND SAGE Foliage of Cleveland sage can be gathered for drying from midsummer into early autumn. Avoid the oldest and youngest leaves, choosing unblemished mature foliage. Dry Cleveland sage as you would common sage (see chapter 4).

Spanish Sage *Salvia lavandulifolia* ZONE 5

Like common sage, Spanish sage grows naturally through much of southern Europe and into northern Africa. Its small, fine-textured, and silvery foliage makes it look a bit like lavender, and indeed it is sometimes called lavender sage. Spanish sage is a variable species, especially when grown from seed. Selected forms are compact and densely branched, while seedlings can be lax and leggy. Garden plants range between a foot and 18 inches in height. Over time, however, this slow spreader may stretch over 3 feet in width, especially when placed on a slightly sloping, sunny hillside.

When handled, the slim, velvety, gray-green leaves release a pungent, penetrating scent that combines the fragrances of common sage and rosemary. This pleasing natural perfume is often used to add depth and resonance to soaps, hand creams, and men's colognes and may be found in aftershaves and antiperspirants. Spanish sage has soft blue flowers on short spikes that are much like those of common sage. Not a heavy bloomer, it is grown chiefly for its beautiful foliage and its traditional medicinal and aromatic properties.

SPANISH SAGE IN THE GARDEN   Well-drained soil and full sun are musts for Spanish sage, which can rot off in heavy soils. It grows best in lean, rather gritty soils that have been lightly amended with compost. In richer soils, Spanish sage has a tendency to develop powdery mildew in dry sites and root rots in damp ones. In less than full sun, even selected forms of Spanish sage can grow leggy and look untidy. In scree conditions (such as a rock garden), this sage tends to be most compact. It does best with no fertilizer other than an annual mulch of aged compost (not more than an inch), and it seldom requires water, except where summers are hot and dry. Periodic deep watering is preferable to constant moisture, which can promote root rots, especially in clay-based soils.

PLEASING PARTNERSHIPS   Evergreen Spanish sage looks particularly handsome in company with other evergreen herbs such as rosemary, lavender, thyme, and common sage. Where winters are mild, it contrasts attractively with shrubby hebes and coppery carexes. Elsewhere, evergreen oat grass (*Helictotrichon sempervirens*) and buttery 'Moonlight' broom (*Cytisus scoparius* 'Moonlight') make excellent companions. A Spanish sage subspecies called *S. l. ssp. blancoana* is especially low growing, making a sprawling, silvery mat of foliage. This tight creeper contrasts well with any evergreen rock plants as well as mats of woolly thyme and small, tufting fescues such as *Festuca amethystina* 'Bronzeglanz'.

GATHERING AND DRYING SPANISH SAGE

Harvest Spanish sage as you would common sage (see chapter 4).

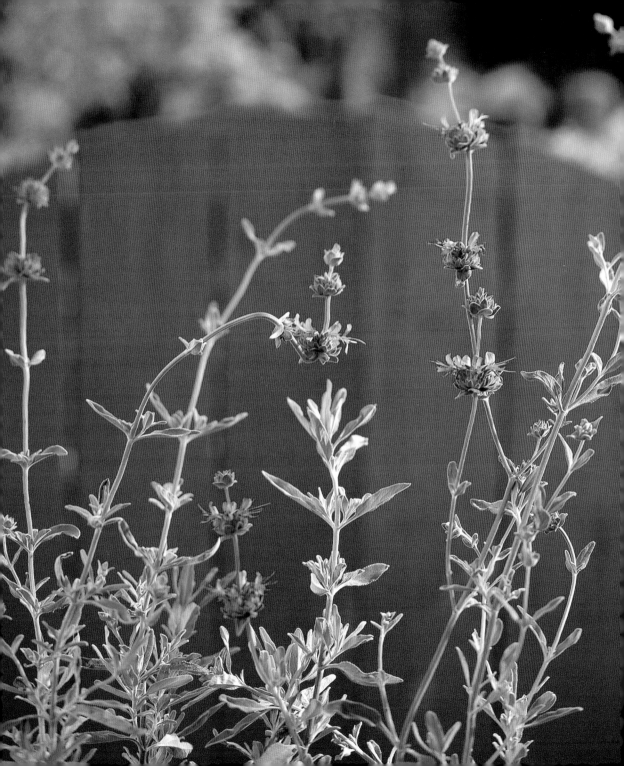

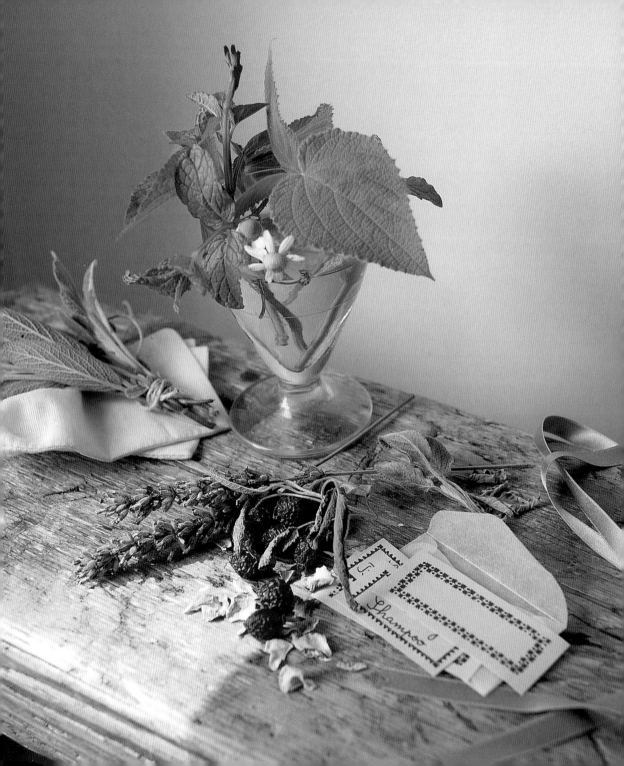

6

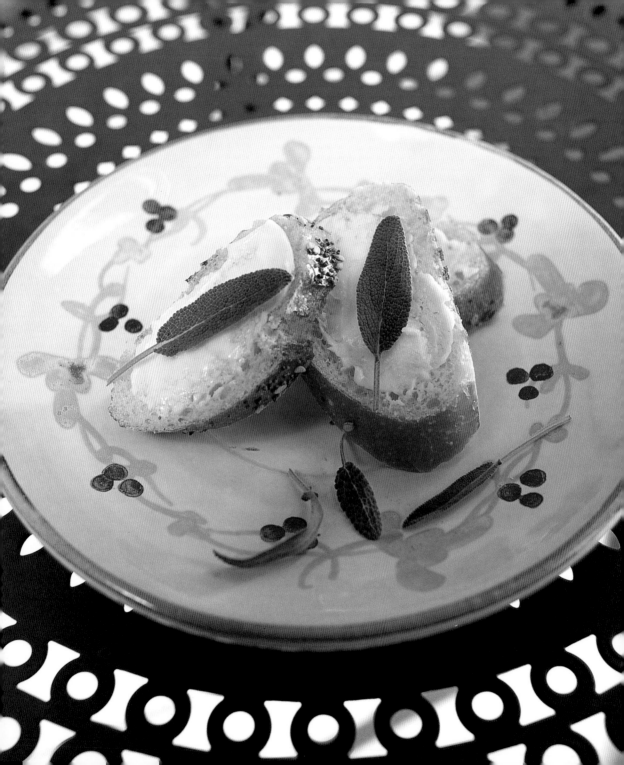

fresh

Few pleasures can rival that of creating delicious, healthy food for family and friends. Somehow even the simplest foods taste even better when they are flavored with our own garden herbs. Fresh or dried foliage and often flowers can add savor to soups, zest to salads, and snap to ordinary sandwiches. A few leaves of common sage turn bread and butter into an elegant appetizer. Shredded fruit sage foliage adds subtle sweetness to fruit salads and gives plain greens a light, citruslike lift. To some people, pineapple sage tastes more like tangerines than pineapples, but however you define it, the complex, sweet-tart flavor works equally well in spicy stir-fries and in sweet fruit smoothies. Clary sage has too much flavor for some taste buds, but those who enjoy its pungent flavor add it to teas and salads as well as soups and stews. Almost everybody finds fried clary sage fritters irresistible (no matter what kind of diet they usually follow).

The recipes you'll find in this chapter are based on four of the most popular culinary salvias: common sage (*S. officinalis*), fruit sage (*S. dorisiana*), pineapple sage (*S. elegans* 'Scarlet Pineapple' and 'Honey Melon'), and clary sage (*S. sclarea*). As you will see, these adaptable herbs can be used in food and drink of all kinds, from appetizers and soups through entrées to desserts.

This recipe sampler begins with an assortment of refreshing teas and tisanes. Some are said to soothe your throat, while others are held to raise your spirits. Most importantly, whatever their putative healing qualities, they should simply taste good. If you find yourself wanting a bit more sweetness or a touch of a sharper, brisker flavor, feel free to add or alter ingredients according to your taste. These classic teas are simply starting places, and any or all may be changed seasonally or even daily.

In my own garden, I like to visit the beds early in the morning with a teapot full of hot water. I enjoy brisk teas in the morning, so I usually begin by combining leaves of common sage with sprigs of lemon thyme and a bit of rosemary. In summer and fall, fruit sage and pineapple sage are frequent contributors to the daily brew. In winter, my calming evening teas generally combine dried fruit sage, mint, and chamomile with a few fresh leaves of common sage.

Common sage is among the most useful herbs in my garden. It's fortunate that constant pinching of the new-growth tips encourages bushy, well-furnished plants, or mine might look decidedly overworked. To avoid stressing my common sage plants by removing too much foliage from any one shrub, I grow over a dozen forms, spacing them throughout the garden.

Since fruit sage and pineapple sage are rarely hardy for me, I grow both in containers. In high summer, when the leaves are at their best, I gather about half the plants for foliage. I always leave a few big clumps for the hummingbirds, which appreciate the late-blooming red flowers. In mild years, I can still gather fresh fruit sage or pineapple sage foliage well into winter. In a hard year, I let the fragrant dried foliage remind me of summer pleasures to come.

Sage in the Kitchen

SAGE TEAS Common sage has a mellow but slightly bitter flavor that most people appreciate when it is combined with other herbs or softened with a bit of honey. Traditionally, sage was used alone for women's tonics and to treat head colds. Sage tea was also used in spring as a blood-cleansing tonic. Village wisewomen often recommended sage tea to bring clarity and wisdom to the troubled spirit.

Traditionally, herb teas are steeped for at least 10 minutes and often longer. Steeping time can considerably alter the way a tea tastes, so if a given tea seems too weak or too strong, simply experiment with varying steeping times and herb amounts to find the intensity you prefer.

NOTE: Pregnant women should restrict sage teas to a single cup per day. While many traditions maintain that sage promotes a comfortable pregnancy and an easy birth, recent research indicates that in rare cases (where underlying conditions already exist), an excessive intake of sage may be deleterious.

Sage Tonic Tea | MAKES 1 CUP

1 tablespoon fresh sage, or 1 teaspoon dried
1 to 2 teaspoons honey

Cover herbs with 1 cup of boiling water, cover, and let steep for 5 to 10 minutes. Strain, add honey to taste, and drink warm or cold.

Wisewoman Sage Tea | MAKES 8 CUPS

This soothing, complex brew smells so good that just sniffing the cup makes you feel better.

- 1 tablespoon fresh sage, or 1 teaspoon dried
- 1 tablespoon fresh fruit sage, or 1 teaspoon dried
- 1 tablespoon fresh pineapple sage, or 1 teaspoon dried
- 1 tablespoon fresh lemon thyme, or 1 teaspoon dried
- 1 tablespoon fresh hops leaves, or 1 teaspoon dried
- 1 tablespoon fresh lemon balm, or 1 teaspoon dried
- 1 tablespoon fresh chamomile, or 1 teaspoon dried
- 1 tablespoon fresh spearmint, or 1 teaspoon dried honey, or to taste

Blend herbs in a mixing bowl. To brew, use 1 tablespoon of fresh herbs or 1 teaspoon of dried herbs per serving. Cover herbs with 1 cup of boiling water per serving, cover, and let steep for 5 to 10 minutes. Strain, add honey, and drink hot, breathing in the aromatic steam.

Heart's Ease Tea | MAKES 4 CUPS

- 1 tablespoon fresh sage, or 1 teaspoon dried
- 1 tablespoon fresh rose petals, or 1 teaspoon dried
- 1 tablespoon fresh chamomile, or 1 teaspoon dried
- 1 tablespoon fresh lemon balm, or 1 teaspoon dried
- Honey (optional)

Blend herbs in a mixing bowl. To brew, use 1 tablespoon of fresh herbs or 1 teaspoon of dried herbs per serving. Cover herbs with 1 cup of boiling water per serving, cover, and let steep for 5 to 10 minutes. Strain, add honey to taste, and drink hot, breathing in the aromatic steam.

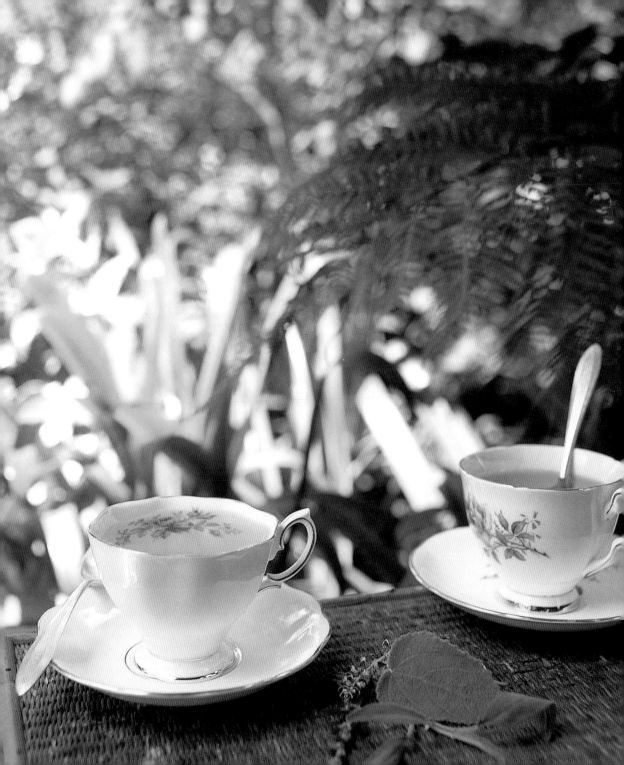

COOKING WITH COMMON SAGE Common sage has long been enjoyed as a rich and savory flavoring for meat and poultry dishes. Turkey stuffing with sage is a classic, but sage is equally enhancing for roasted chicken or pork. Simply loosening the skin of any game bird and tucking in fresh sage leaves will add a subtle, smoky piquancy to the simplest roast fowl. In Italy and France, a traditional healing sage soup was served after an illness and early in the New Year to promote good health. Chopped sage and a bit of rosemary enlivens any soup. Indeed, the addition of a teaspoon or two of minced herbs at heating time can even make a store-bought soup taste freshly made.

Fresh sage leaves also bring a pleasing warmth and depth of flavor to plain salads and ordinary sandwiches. Good alone, common sage is especially delicious in combination with other fresh herbs. Try adding shredded sage and lemon balm to your usual recipe for tuna sandwiches, or toss slivered sage leaves with basil, chives, and silver mint into a garden salad of tomatoes, sweet peppers, and cucumbers.

Sage canapés complement any salad or soup and are an excellent foil for good wines. The secret of this exceedingly simple recipe is to use excellent bread and butter and to pick middle-sized sage leaves, choosing neither the youngest nor the most mature. Look for leaves that are uniformly silvery in coloring, rather than mottled older foliage. Following, you will find a selection of other recipes to spark your kitchen creativity.

Roast Chicken with Common Sage | SERVES 4

    1 whole roasting chicken
    3 to 4 cloves garlic, peeled
    ¼ cup fresh common sage leaves
    1 onion, coarsely chopped
    1 teaspoon salt

Rinse chicken and pat dry. Cut each clove of garlic into 5 or 6 thick slices. With a sharp paring knife, puncture chicken skin and flesh, making 1-inch cuts a few inches apart. Insert a slice of garlic in each cut. Next, insert 12 or so whole sage leaves into the cuts, sliding the leaves completely under the skin so they lie flat against the flesh. Toss remaining sage with onion and salt and stuff chicken cavity loosely. Bake chicken at 350° F until juices run clear and skin is crisp and golden brown (about an hour).

Saltimbocca | SERVES 4

  1 pound veal round, thinly sliced (about 8 slices)
  $\frac{1}{4}$ pound prosciutto, thinly sliced (about 8 slices)
  16 fresh sage leaves
  4 tablespoons butter
  2 tablespoons olive oil
  kosher or sea salt
  freshly ground pepper
  4 sprigs sage
  1 lemon, cut in wedges

Preheat oven to 200° F and put a serving platter in the oven to warm. Gently pound veal to flatten each piece. Trim pieces of prosciutto to fit over veal. Place 2 sage leaves on each piece of veal and top with prosciutto. Roll veal so prosciutto is enclosed and pin shut with a toothpick. Melt 2 tablespoons butter with oil in a large frying pan over medium-high heat. Sprinkle veal lightly with kosher salt and pepper. Cook veal in hot butter, turning as soon as the edges of the veal turn white. When cooked on all sides (about 2 to 3 minutes per piece), remove veal to warm platter. Add remaining butter to pan and deglaze, scraping off crisp bits. Pour hot butter over veal and serve at once, garnished with sage sprigs and lemon wedges.

Gnocchi with Sage Butter | SERVES 4

12 leaves fresh common sage
2 tablespoons sweet butter
3 to 4 tablespoons fruity olive oil
2 to 3 cloves garlic, peeled and mashed
1 teaspoon kosher salt
¼ cup walnuts, toasted
1 pound fresh or frozen gnocchi
pepper to taste

Mince 1 tablespoon fresh sage and blend with sweet butter. Set aside. In a saucepan, heat oil over medium-low heat with whole, mashed garlic cloves and 2 tablespoons coarsely chopped common sage leaves. Sprinkle with 1 teaspoon salt. Brown garlic lightly on both sides; then discard cloves, add walnuts, and reduce heat to lowest setting. Cook gnocchi according to directions on package; drain and arrange in four bowls. Drizzle with sage-infused oil and serve at once, garnished with sage butter, fresh sage, and freshly ground pepper.

Sage Baked New Potatoes | SERVES 4

1 pound red-skinned new potatoes
1 to 2 tablespoons olive oil
¼ cup fresh common sage leaves
kosher salt

Preheat oven to 350° F. Scrub new potatoes and cut in halves. Cover a 9-by-13-inch baking dish with a thin coating of oil and arrange sage leaves over the entire surface. Sprinkle with salt and arrange potatoes on the leaves, placing them cut-side down. Bake for 1 hour at 350° F or about 90 minutes at 325° F. Serve warm.

French Sage Soup | SERVES 2

12 fresh common sage leaves, shredded
1 teaspoon salt
1 teaspoon pepper
1 tablespoon olive oil
1 small onion, chopped coarsely
2 slices crusty bread
2 tablespoons grated hard cheese (asiago, pecorino, or Parmesan)

Combine sage, ½ teaspoon salt, and ½ teaspoon pepper with 2 cups boiling water. Cover and steep for 10 minutes. In a saucepan heat 2 teaspoons olive oil over medium-high heat. Add onion, stir well to coat, and sprinkle with salt and pepper. When onion is soft and pale golden, add sage infusion (leaves included). Simmer for 10 minutes. While soup simmers, spread remaining olive oil on bread. Sprinkle with one-half the cheese and toast until crisp. When soup is hot through, adjust seasoning (salt and pepper to taste) and serve hot with cheese toast, garnishing soup with remaining cheese.

Sage Canapés | MAKES 2 DOZEN

24 fresh common sage leaves
24 small (2-inch) rounds French baguette or any crusty bread
sweet butter
kosher salt

Rinse sage and pat dry. Spread bread rounds with butter and sprinkle lightly with salt. Set a sage leaf on each and serve at room temperature.

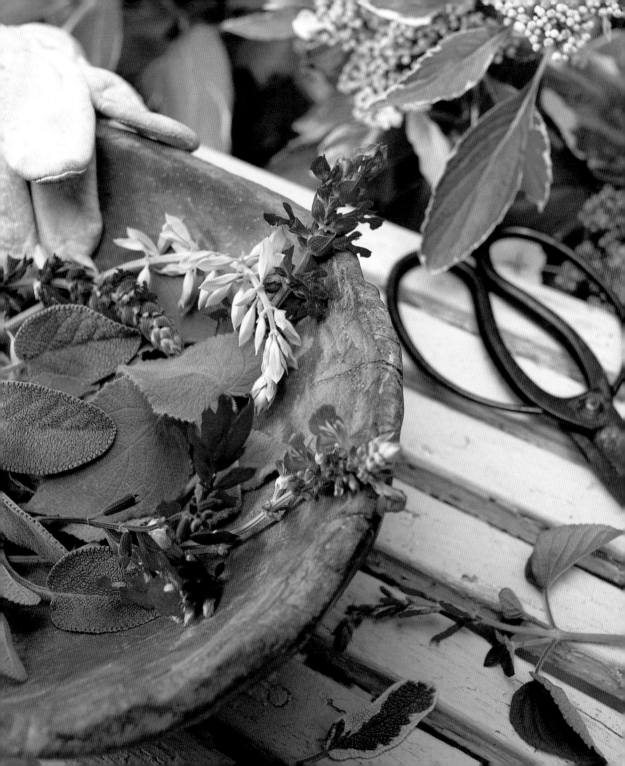

Fruit Sage in the Kitchen

Mild and sweet in flavor, shredded fruit sage foliage is an adaptable herb that can be employed in either sweet or savory dishes. Fresh foliage is especially tasty when added generously to salads. A simple base of young greens can be enriched with poached chicken, shredded fruit sage, and lemon balm. Enliven a mixture of plain greens with the tingling bite of arugula and a bit of bitter radicchio, then toss in stir-fried shrimp with shredded fruit sage and cilantro. Spritz on some fresh lime juice, a sprinkle of kosher salt, and lots of pepper for a quick and fiery feast.

Fruit sage is delightful in cold soups of almost any kind. Shredded leaves add a delicate tang to chilled Scandinavian cherry soups. Minced together with dill and chives, the foliage will lend a soft, almost floral brightness to a creamy shrimp bisque. Chopped fruit sage and mint will wake up yogurt-based cucumber soups and mild curries.

This easygoing herb combines especially well with herbs that are full flavored but not overpowering. Chives, lemon balm, lemon thyme, sweet basil, and silver mint or butter mint are all excellent companions for fruit sage, as are chamomile and lemon grass. If you use fruit sage with fruit, try adding a sprinkle of fructose instead of regular sugar. Fructose or fruit sugar potentiates the flavor of fresh fruits and sweet herbs. You'll find you can use less fructose than regular sugar while getting a fuller, sweeter fruity flavor.

Fruit Sage Iced Tea | MAKES 4 CUPS

¼ cup fresh fruit sage foliage

2 tablespoons fresh chamomile flowers

2 tablespoons fresh lemon balm

2 tablespoons fresh silver mint or spearmint

1 tablespoon green tea

2 teaspoons fructose or 1 tablespoon honey

Combine herbs with green tea and stir to blend. Add 4 cups boiling water and steep, covered, for 3 to 5 minutes (to taste). Strain mixture and taste, diluting as desired and adding fructose or honey to taste while mixture is hot. Serve chilled. Freeze any leftovers as ice cubes to use with lemonade or iced tea.

Fruit Sage and Ginger Sorbet | SERVES 4 *to* 6

2 cups sugar or 1 ⅓ cup fructose
¼ cup fruit sage leaves, shredded
2 to 3 inches of ginger root, peeled and minced (2 to 3 tablespoons)
grated zest of 1 large organic lemon
about ¼ cup fresh lemon juice

In a heavy saucepan, combine sugar or fructose, fruit sage, ginger, and 1 teaspoon grated lemon zest with 4 cups water and bring to a boil over medium-high heat, stirring often. Reduce heat to medium and simmer, uncovered, for 10 minutes. Cool mixture; then add lemon juice, stirring well. Freeze in an ice cream maker or in an ice cube tray until solid (about 6 hours). Put serving bowl in freezer to chill. Whirl frozen cubes in a blender or food processor until smooth, transfer to chilled serving bowl, and freeze until firm (about an hour). Serve cold.

Summery Fruit Salad with Fruit Sage Dressing | SERVES 4

1 cup peaches, peeled and sliced
1 cup blueberries
1 cup raspberries
1 cup cantaloupe, cut into balls or ½-inch cubes
1 tablespoon fructose or sugar
2 to 3 teaspoons lime juice
1 cup yogurt (nonfat works fine)
grated zest of 1 organic lime
2 tablespoons honey
2 tablespoons fresh fruit sage foliage, shredded
few drops vanilla
2 to 3 sprigs fruit sage for garnish

Combine fruit in a serving bowl. Sprinkle with fructose or sugar and lime juice, and toss gently. In a smaller bowl, combine yogurt with 1 teaspoon grated lime zest, honey, fruit sage, and vanilla. Stir well, pour over fruit, garnish and serve at once.

Pineapple Sage in the Kitchen

Pineapple sage is especially effective where its zesty, citruslike quality is showcased, as in sorbets, teas, and lemonades. As with fruit sage, you'll find that fructose (fruit sugar) enhances flavor more than table sugar or honey. A little fructose goes a long way in fruit-flavored treats, so begin with less than your usual amount of sugar and taste as you go.

Fresh or dried, pineapple sage foliage adds zip to fruit- or vegetable-based cold soups, sauces, and spreads. For a quick dip, blend chopped pineapple sage, mint, and lemon balm into a cup of hummus. Minced with marjoram and chives, pineapple sage adds sparkle and sweetness to sandwiches filled with curried chicken or smoked salmon salads.

For a refreshing main dish, serve grilled chicken on a bed of fresh, shredded pineapple sage and French sorrel. A handful of minced leaves and a spoonful of capers turn chilled, grilled salmon into a sprightly snack or light entrée. Sizzle lean, fast-cooking pork medallions with garlic, ginger, and pineapple sage and serve over hot rice.

Pineapple sage makes a tasty addition to salads and sandwiches. Add minced pineapple sage to a vinaigrette made from sweet rice vinegar and a soft, fruity olive oil to dress buttery baby spinach tossed with fresh goat cheese and slivered Florence fennel. For a quick garden salad dressing, blend shredded pineapple sage with grated carrots, golden raisins, and walnuts with yogurt or sour cream (nonfat works fine) and a splash of balsamic vinegar.

Pineapple Sage Smoothie | SERVES 4

    1 banana, cut in chunks
    1 cup honeydew or any melon, cubed
    1 cup raspberries
    1 cup strawberries, trimmed and cut in half
    ¼ cup pineapple sage leaves, shredded
    2 teaspoons fructose or honey
    4 cups yogurt (nonfat works fine)
    1 teaspoon vanilla

Combine all ingredients in a blender or food processor and blend to desired consistency. Serve immediately (at room temperature) for fullest flavor.

Curried Chicken Salad with Honey Melon Sage Dressing | SERVES 4

2 cups yogurt or sour cream (nonfat works fine)

2 tablespoons 'Honey Melon' or pineapple sage foliage, shredded

2 tablespoons silver mint or spearmint, shredded

1 clove garlic, minced

$\frac{1}{2}$ teaspoon kosher or sea salt

1 to 2 teaspoons tikka or sweet curry powder

2 cups cooked chicken, cut in $\frac{1}{2}$-inch pieces

$\frac{1}{4}$ cup dried apricots, cut in 3 or 4 slices

2 tablespoons dry Marsala or balsamic vinegar

2 stalks celery, thinly sliced

1 'Gypsy Fiesta' or any red bell pepper, thinly sliced

$\frac{1}{4}$ cup peanuts

4 sprigs pineapple sage foliage and flower (if available)

In a medium bowl, combine yogurt or sour cream with shredded herbs, garlic, salt, and curry powder. Let sit for 15 minutes; then taste and adjust seasoning (salt and curry powder) to taste. Set aside. In a small bowl, combine chicken, apricots, and dry Marsala or balsamic vinegar. Cover with waxed paper and heat in microwave for 1 minute (or heat wine or vinegar to a simmer; then pour over the chicken and apricots). Let steep, covered, for 5 to 10 minutes until apricots take up most of the liquid. In a larger bowl, toss chicken mixture with celery and bell pepper, set aside. When apricots are plumped, drain off excess liquid and toss with chicken mixture. Gently stir in yogurt mixture and serve at once, garnished with peanuts and pineapple sage foliage and flowers.

Pineapple Sage Sorbet | SERVES 4 *to* 6

2 cups sugar or 1 ⅓ cups fructose
¼ cup pineapple sage leaves, shredded
grated zest of 1 large organic lemon
about ¼ cup fresh lemon juice

In a heavy saucepan, combine sugar or fructose, sage, and 2 teaspoons grated lemon zest with 4 cups water and bring to a boil over medium-high heat, stirring often. Reduce heat to medium and simmer, uncovered, for 10 minutes. Cool mixture; then add lemon juice and freeze in an ice cream maker or in an ice cube tray until solid (about 6 hours). Put serving bowl in freezer to chill. Whirl frozen cubes in a blender or food processor until smooth, transfer to chilled serving bowl, and freeze until firm (about an hour). Serve cold.

Clary Sage in the Kitchen

Clary sage has many traditional medicinal uses, from eye treatments to healing teas and tisanes. Tisanes are French herbal teas, hot or cold infusions of herbs with water, wine, or other liquids. The word comes from the Greek phrase for crushed barley and refers to an ancient, medicinal, cooling drink made from sage and grains.

One popular winter tisane, often used to treat colds and flus, combined sage leaves, thyme, and rosehips. This tasty drink does indeed feel soothing when you are ill, and the natural antiseptic qualities of sage and thyme and the vitamin c of rosehips may indeed confer some benefit.

In Germany, local Rhine wines were often mulled with clary sage and elder flowers (*Sambucus nigra*) to lend them the floral scent of a good Muscadet (muscat wine). The sage-infused wine not only smells and tastes great but was also traditionally held to have healing properties. A small glass after dinner was prescribed for those recovering from fevers, long illness, or physical or emotional exhaustion, and was a popular ladies' tonic.

Another version of this old favorite is made like May wine, traditionally a light wine flavored with sweet woodruff blossoms. To make a summery clary sage spritzer, add minced fresh foliage and a few blossoms to any sweet white wine. For starters, try a spicy Riesling or Gewürztraminer, though a flowery rosé would also be suitable.

Clary Sage and Rosehip Tisane | MAKES 2 CUPS

2 tablespoons fresh clary sage leaves, or 1 tablespoon dried
2 tablespoons fresh thyme leaves, or 1 tablespoon dried
2 tablespoons fresh rosehips, or 1 tablespoon dried
honey

Combine herbs and rosehips in a culinary herb bag (or simply place in a small saucepan). Add 2 cups boiling water, cover, and let steep for 15 minutes. Remove herb bag or strain and return liquid to pan. Over medium-high heat, bring tisane to a slow simmer (2 to 3 minutes). Add honey to taste and serve hot.

Clary Sage Mulled Wine | SERVES 6 *to* 8

2 tablespoons fresh clary sage leaves, or 1 tablespoon dried
2 tablespoons fresh European elder flowers (*Sambucus nigra*),
    or 1 tablespoon dried
honey (optional)
1 bottle red wine (any kind, though German Rhine wines are traditional)

Put sage leaves and elder flowers in a culinary herb bag. Place herb bag in a saucepan with the wine and bring to a simmer over medium-low heat. Do not boil. Steep mixture over lowest heat for 10 to 20 minutes (to taste). Remove herbs or strain wine and serve hot, adding honey to taste if desired.

Clary Sage Fritters | MAKES ABOUT 3 DOZEN

    1 egg, lightly beaten
    1 cup flour
    kosher salt
    2 to 3 tablespoons milk
    oil for frying
    6 clary sage leaves, cut in 2-by-2-inch pieces

Blend egg, flour, and ½ teaspoon salt in a mixing bowl, adding milk as needed to make a thin batter; then let stand. Heat about ¾-inch oil in a heavy frying pan over medium-high heat. When oil is hot, dip leaves in batter and fry in oil until crisp and golden brown, turning once. Lightly sprinkle each piece with kosher salt and drain on paper towels. Serve warm.

Clary Sage Vinegar | MAKES 2 CUPS

    2 cups red wine vinegar
    2 tablespoons fresh clary sage leaf, shredded
    1 teaspoon fresh rosemary

Warm vinegar over medium-low heat (do not boil). Add herbs, remove from heat, then cover and let steep for 1 hour. Strain into a jar or bottle, adding a sprig of rosemary for garnish if desired. Store out of direct sunlight.

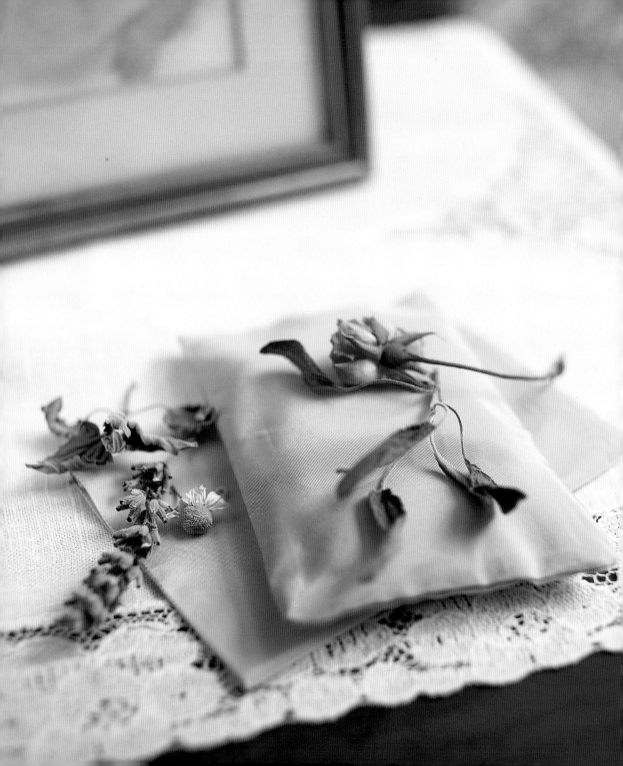

colorful

This final section presents you with a different kind of recipe. In the following pages, you'll learn how to create all sorts of herbal delights, from simple hand creams and homemade shampoos to herb-filled bath bags and stimulating facial steams. Most of the recipes and techniques presented here are simple, and though some products need time to blend or mellow, few require more than a few minutes of effort.

If you enjoy these introductory activities, you may decide to explore this fascinating field in further depth. If so, you will find a list of manuals, handbooks, and guides to crafting with herbs in "Sources and Resources" at the end of this book.

Though many of the ingredients can be grown at home, others, like essential oils, can be costly. In part this reflects the fact that significant quantities of fresh herbs are required to make even modest amounts of these oils. Then, too, essential oil extraction devices are quite expensive. Such an investment can quickly turn an inexpensive hobby into an extremely expensive one.

If you are handy with a sewing machine, you can save yourself a fair amount of money by making, rather than buying, culinary and bath herbal bags. These come in handy when sage leaves and other herbs are soaked in wine or made into teas, since putting foliage into a culinary herb bag eliminates straining and saves cleanup time. These small cotton drawstring bags can be bought at many culinary supply shops. If you can't find them, they can be made from muslin or any coarse, open-weave cotton material by following the directions for making herbal bath bags offered in the section on crafting with fruit sage (page 120).

In most cases, you can experiment freely with these basic recipes, adding herbs that you enjoy smelling. However, be aware that certain herbs, such as rue (*Ruta graveolens*), can cause skin irritations. Not everyone is equally sensitive, but you don't want to find out the hard way. Before you use an herb not mentioned in the text, please check with your local poison control or look it up in one of the herbal reference works listed in "Sources and Resources" at the end of this book.

Sage for Health and Beauty

As we have seen, common sage has many traditional uses, including a plenitude of healing mixtures. Among the simplest are the gargles, rinses for sore mouths and throats. If you don't enjoy the deep flavor of common sage, you can amplify the basic recipe with other healing herbs such as thyme and rosemary. Both of these serviceable herbs are said to have mild antiseptic properties similar to those of common sage, and many people find their flavors pleasing. Lemon thyme tastes soft and citrusy, while the extra-hardy 'Arp' rosemary has a milder, gentler flavor than brisk pine-scented kinds.

Common sage is also said to ease strained or pulled muscles and to help relax those that are tight and sore from overwork. Following, you'll find a relaxing, bath-salt blend that once again combines common sage with mint, rosemary, and thyme. In summer, I often add a little fruit sage to the mix for extra sparkle and fragrance. Unscented bath salts can be found in bulk at many health stores and pharmacies. To brighten up your home-made bath-salt mixtures, you can also mix in dried petals of vividly colorful flowers like calendulas and violets to make confetti-colored blends.

Dream pillows are an old folk tradition that is enjoying a new surge in popularity these days. Serious dream-pillow makers insist that each herb has its particular meaning and properties that can affect the way we sleep as well as our dreams. All of the ingredients used in the dream-pillow recipe given on page 118—common sage, hops, valerian, and catnip—are commonly considered to be soothing, sleep-inducing, and productive of pleasant dreams.

Sage Throat Gargle

$\frac{1}{4}$ cup fresh common sage leaves
2 tablespoons fresh rosemary
1 tablespoon fresh chamomile flowers

Combine herbs with 1 cup boiling water; then cover and steep for 20 minutes. Strain and refrigerate in tightly closed jar. Use as a mouthwash or throat gargle. Keeps for 2 weeks in refrigerator.

Sage Bath Salts for Sore Muscles

3 tablespoons dried common sage leaves
1 tablespoon dried rosemary leaves
1 tablespoon dried mint
1 tablespoon dried thyme
1 cup sea salt or unscented bath salts

Combine all herbs and grind together coarsely with a mortar and pestle, or crumble with the hands into a coarse powder. Combine with salt, stirring well to blend. Store in a tightly sealed jar. To use, add 2 to 3 tablespoons to a bathtub full of hot water.

Sage in Dream Pillows

Dream pillows are small sachets of dried herbs used to promote relaxation and sweet dreams. Tucked under a pillow, the fragrant herbs create a natural perfume that can pleasantly affect your night's sleep. Here's a traditional dream-pillow mixture using common sage, thought to bring healing wisdom to troubled dreamers.

2 tablespoons dried common sage foliage
2 tablespoons dried hops bracts
2 tablespoons dried valerian foliage
2 tablespoons dried catnip foliage
2 tablespoons dried chamomile flowers
2 tablespoons dried rose petals
2 tablespoons dried rosemary
2 tablespoons dried lavender

Blend all ingredients in a mixing bowl and divide between two small cotton sachet bags. Sew bags shut. If desired, cover dream pillows with small slipcovers of smooth cotton. Makes 1 cup of mixture, enough for two dream pillows.

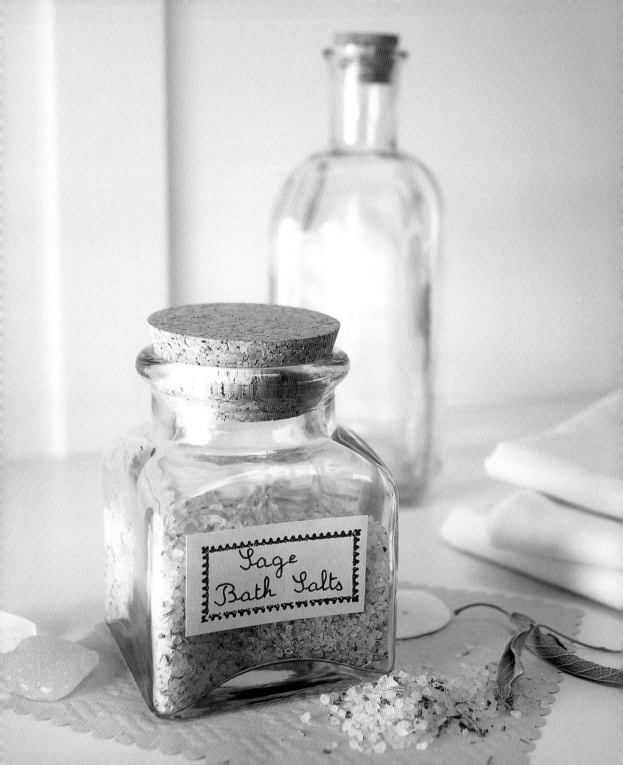

Fruit Sage for Health and Beauty

Fruit sage is said to have skin-softening properties and to be an effective cleansing herb for the skin. Here it adds its soft, subtle perfume to a creamy, easily made hand lotion that softens as it scents. In different proportions the same basic ingredients can be combined to make an enticing herbal bath blend.

The simple baseline recipes presented in the following pages will make a good starting place for your own exploration with healing herbal mixtures. But many of these recipes are not just introductory: they are simple because simple things often work very well. A cup of plain fruit sage foliage can turn an ordinary bath into a tropical adventure all on its own. Play freely with your own herbal bath blends, using all sorts of scents that appeal to you (keeping in mind the precaution that some herbs like rue can irritate sensitive skin).

For relaxing baths, combine fragrant flowers such as jasmine, honeysuckle, and rose petals with sweet-scented herbs like chocolate mint, lemon balm, and chamomile. To enjoy a more invigorating experience, try adding small amounts of more pungent herbs such as common sage, lemon thyme, lavender, and rosemary.

To avoid clogging your drain, use herbal bath bags, which are sold in many herb supply stores. If you can't find any, they may be made from muslin or any loosely woven cotton material.

For use with small quantities of mulling or tea herbs, you can scale down the finished bag by a third, making it closer to the size of a traditional tea bag. To avoid losing a lot of liquid to absorption, wet the bag thoroughly with water after adding the herbs but before placing it in the wine or tea liquid.

To avoid clogging your drain, use herbal bath bags, which are sold in many herb supply stores. If you can't find any, they can be made from muslin or any loosely woven cotton material.

MAKING HERBAL BATH BAGS To make a long-lasting herbal bath bag, cut a rectangle of cloth twice the desired size, adding an inch to each side for seam allowance. Sew the bag closed on the two long sides, leaving an open neck. Fold over the raw edges of the neck so they are on the same side as the seams, and then hem each edge, leaving a 1-inch channel for the drawstring. Reverse bag so seams are on the inside, and thread the drawstring channel with about 18 inches of light cord.

Fruit Sage Hand Lotion

$\frac{1}{4}$ cup fresh fruit sage foliage
2 tablespoons fresh lemon balm
2 tablespoons fresh lavender
2 tablespoons fresh rose petals
$\frac{1}{2}$ cup glycerin

Cover herbs with 1 cup boiling water; cover and let steep for 20 minutes. Strain herbs through a sieve, pushing with the back of a spoon or squeezing with your hands to remove all liquid from leaves. Slowly blend strained liquid into $\frac{1}{2}$ cup of glycerin, stirring well. Store in a tightly closed jar out of direct sunlight. To use, rub a small amount into hands after washing. Glycerin must be fresh or lotion will be very thin. For thicker lotion, increase the amount of glycerin until the desired consistency is achieved.

Fruit Sage Herbal Bath

$\frac{1}{4}$ cup fresh fruit sage foliage
1 tablespoon fresh lemon balm
1 teaspoon fresh lavender
1 teaspoon fresh rose petals

Combine all ingredients in a bowl and stir well. Place herbs in a drawstring mesh bag large enough to hold the herbs without compacting them (generally about 4 by 6 inches). To use, toss in a bathtub full of hot water.

Pineapple Sage for Health and Beauty

A relatively recent introduction to North America gardeners, pineapple sage is already quite common in our gardens. It ought to be a frequent visitor in the kitchen as well, for the big leaves of this easy-to-grow salvia are deliciously fragrant, even more so than the hot red flowers, whose scent is both softer and less penetrating.

Below you'll find a number of quickly prepared recipes that take advantage of the bright, frisky scent of pineapple sage foliage. As always, you can make a more intensely perfumed product by adding rose petals and other fragrant flowers as well as aromatic herbs that please your nose. Don't, however, leave out any ingredients, because all of the listed herbs play an active role in making these mixtures effective. For instance, fresh or dried pineapple sage leaves add their citrusy sweetness to an herbal hair rinse that leaves the hair soft and shiny. However, the real work is being done by common sage, rosemary, and chamomile, all of which help to soften and strengthen hair.

Pineapple sage also lends its fruity perfume to my favorite shampoo, the one I swear by and use daily. For gardeners who spend lots of time outside, this shampoo can help bring dried-out hair back to glossy health. Here again, the working herbs are common sage, rosemary, and chamomile.

You can use any mild, unscented shampoo or Castile-type soap for the base of home-made shampoos. I prefer to start with a pure Castile liquid soap like Dr. Bronner's Baby Mild. This widely available brand uses natural rosemary extract as a preservative and antioxidant.

Pineapple Sage Hair-Rinse

¼ cup fresh pineapple sage, or 2 tablespoons dried
2 tablespoons fresh chamomile flowers, or 1 tablespoon dried
2 tablespoons fresh rosemary, or 1 tablespoon dried
2 tablespoons fresh common sage, or 1 tablespoon dried

Cover herbs with 2 cups boiling water, cover, and steep for 20 minutes. Strain herbs through a sieve, pushing with the back of a spoon to remove all liquid from leaves. Use fresh or store in a tightly covered jar in the refrigerator for up to a week. To use, pour ½ cup of herbal rinse over freshly washed, wet hair. Towel dry; then brush out hair while still damp. To control curly hair, brush while damp, let dry for 5 minutes, and then push gently to set smooth water waves.

Three-Sage Shampoo

1 tablespoon dried pineapple sage
1 tablespoon dried common sage
1 tablespoon dried fruit sage
1 tablespoon dried chamomile flowers
1 tablespoon dried rosemary
8 ounces liquid Castile soap (with peppermint if plain is unavailable)
   or 8 ounces baby shampoo

Place herbs in a saucepan and cover with 1 cup boiling water. Cover and steep for 20 minutes. Strain herbs through a sieve, pushing with the back of a spoon to remove all liquid from leaves. Slowly pour Castile soap or baby shampoo into herbal liquid while still hot, stirring well to blend. Store in tightly capped squeeze bottle. Shake well before each use.

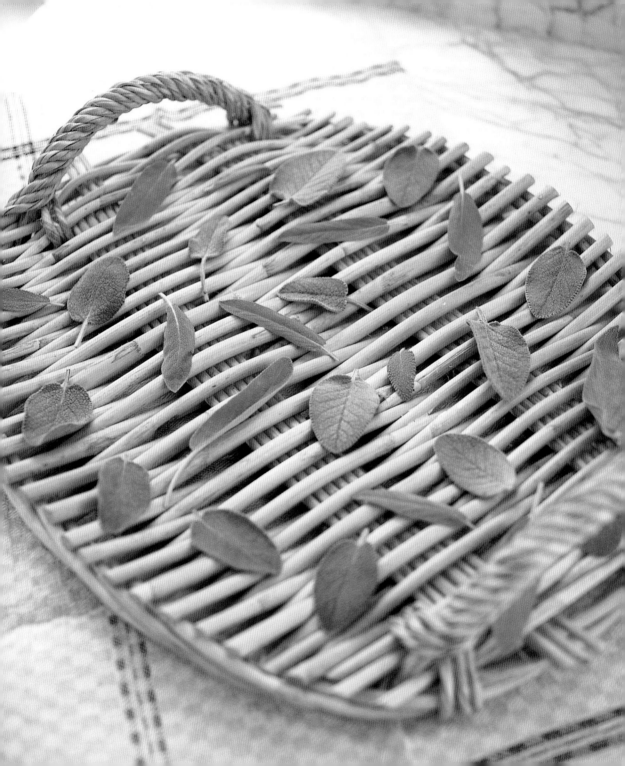

Clary Sage for Health and Beauty

Like common sage, clary sage has traditional uses that range from the kitchen to the altar. In Europe, over-the-counter eye drops often contain clary sage extract to clarify tired eyes. (They are also apt to contain belladonna or deadly nightshade as well, a potent and poisonous drug that makes the user's eyes look especially bright and shiny. Do not try this at home.) A teaspoon of dried clary sage added to your morning tea is also said to make your eyes look brighter. I don't know if this really does anything cosmetic for one's eyes, but it certainly makes your tea smell good.

During the Dark Ages and in medieval times, clary-sage smudges were used to bring healing smoke to patients suffering from serious diseases. The simple, unbound sage smudge described below was widely used in England and Europe until quite recent times (England's Regency period) to purify sickroom air after any lengthy illness. For more information about using clary sages in the bundled sage smudges made for traditional ceremonial use, see the sidebar on smudge making on page 63.

Double-Sage Sickroom Smudge

12 leaves dried common sage
3 leaves dried clary sage, cut in several pieces

Put dried leaves into a sturdy, fireproof ashtray or saucer and light with a candle or long, fireplace match. Sage leaves ignite and burn slowly, creating a light, aromatic smoke. Let the leaves burn completely (you may need to relight them once or twice). Leave the room closed for 24 hours; then air out completely (open all windows for at least a few hours or overnight).

Cleveland Sage for Health and Beauty

This beautiful and intensely fragrant California native has been associated with smudging and purification ceremonies for centuries. The dried leaves and twigs can be used alone or in combination with cedar and wild desert sages (artemisias) to make bundled ceremonial cleansing smudges. Since Cleveland sage dries out very quickly, these are best made with fresh material. When they are freshly gathered, handling the leaves is an active pleasure. Once dry, both leaves and stems become brittle and shatter easily.

For a simpler room-cleansing effect, put a cupful of fresh, Cleveland sage leaves into a shallow bowl and observe how they gradually fill even a large room with their rich, sparkling scent. Though it is only one of many ingredients in the potpourri mixture described below, the subtle, tantalizing fragrance of Cleveland sage provides the dominant note. Over time, it adds increasing depth to the perfume.

Cleveland Sage Potpourri

    1 cup dried Cleveland sage foliage
    1 cup dried rose petals
    1 cup dried lavender leaves and flowers
    1 cup dried sweet Annie (*Artemisia annua*) foliage
    2-inch section of a vanilla bean
    2 tablespoons dried rosemary foliage
    1 tablespoon dried orange zest
    1 tablespoon ground orris root (fixative)
    2 to 3 drops clary sage oil
    2 to 3 drops rose oil

Toss dried leaves and flowers gently (like a salad). Add orange zest and orris root and stir carefully to blend. Dot essential oils over the whole and shake gently. Store in an oversized, tightly closed jar or container (mixture should fill container about halfway) for 6 to 8 weeks, shaking container once or twice a week while melding. To use, put ½ cup of mixture into a bowl and set in a room that needs refreshing, or use in sachets. Store remaining mixture in tightly covered jar out of direct light.

Spanish Sage for Health and Beauty

Spanish sage is notably free with its fragrance in the garden. It also lends its penetrating and refreshing perfume to a number of commercial products for skin and hair care. In this section, you will find a recipe for a stimulating facial masque, a simple herbal treatment that leaves the face feeling silky soft and deeply clean. This masque works best when the skin pores are already open, so try it while you soak in a long, hot bath.

Spanish sage foliage also contributes healing properties to the soothing hand lotion and amplifies its clean, light fragrance. Like thyme, many salvias (including this one) have natural antiseptic properties. This homemade hand lotion is especially useful for gardeners, whose hands can be hard to clean and whose scratches can easily get infected. The recipe on page 128 is one of several similar recipes that were field-tested by the Friday Tidy team, a group of volunteer gardeners who maintain award-winning gardens at the public library on Bainbridge Island, Washington. This was their pick for the best lotion to use before donning garden gloves.

Spanish Sage Facial Masque

2 teaspoons fresh Spanish sage foliage, or 1 teaspoon dried

2 teaspoons fresh elder flowers, or 1 teaspoon dried

2 teaspoons fresh lemon balm, or 1 teaspoon dried

2 teaspoons fresh butter mint or spearmint, or 1 teaspoon dried

2 tablespoons colloidal oatmeal (bath oats)

Blend all ingredients, stirring well. Add 3 to 4 tablespoons boiling water; cover and steep for 10 minutes. Mixture will be a thick paste (adjust with hot water to spreadable thickness as needed). To use, first wash face with warm water; then dip washcloth into very hot water, wring it out, and cover face for 10 seconds. Remove cloth and evenly apply warm paste to face, scrubbing lightly. Leave lips, nostrils, and eye areas uncovered. Let dry and then rinse off with warm water.

Spanish Sage Gardener's Hand Cream

¼ cup olive, almond, or grapeseed oil

¼ cup fresh Spanish sage foliage, or 2 tablespoons dried

2 tablespoons fresh lemon thyme (or any thyme), or 1 tablespoon dried

2 tablespoons calendula gel (available at health-food stores)

1 cup wax-based, unscented skin cream such as Eucerin (available at pharmacies)

Warm oil over low heat (do not boil). Add herbs; then remove from heat and steep, covered, for an hour. Strain, discard herbs, and blend oil into calendula gel, stirring well. Slowly add skin cream, a spoonful at a time, blending well before each addition. Store in a tightly closed jar out of direct light. To use, apply generously to hands before putting on garden gloves and again, more sparingly, after gardening.

Creating, Storing, and Using Sage Oils

Volatile or essential oils are natural plant oils that carry fragrance and flavor in their foliage and stems, roots, and bark. Unlike fixed oils (such as olive oil and walnut oil), essential oils evaporate readily, which makes them difficult to extract and store. Highly concentrated essential oils are very potent in scent and flavor and are used sparingly, a drop at a time. To preserve their special properties (which vary from plant to plant), essential oils are stored in dark-colored, tightly stoppered bottles to protect them from the degrading effects of light and air.

Unless you have access to a chemistry lab, the most practical way for a home herbalist to make essential oil is with a steam distiller. These devices use steam from boiling water to remove essential oils from herb foliage. The steam is then cooled in a condenser to concentrate the oil. Because oils are lighter than water, they can be removed from the surface of the cooled steam (water) with a long-necked glass eyedropper.

It takes a lot of herb foliage to make even a small amount of essential oil. Depending on the herb involved, you can expect to get about an ounce of essential oil from 1 or 2 quarts of fresh foliage. To get the most from your herbs, harvest the leaves when the flowers begin to bud up. After the flowers bloom, the quantity of essential oil in the foliage is reduced. However, you will still get a fair amount of essential oil even if you harvest after the plant is in bloom.

If you want to make a pure essential oil, use foliage from a single kind of plant, such as common sage. If you want to make a lively mixture, you can make a blend of scented herbs such as sage, rosemary, lavender, and thyme by combining the foliage in your steam unit. This is a great way to use up trimmings of herb plants that need summer shaping or cutting back. The fragrant result can be used in soaps and lotions, added (drop by drop) to potpourri and dream pillow mixtures, or used to scent candles.

Small steam distilling units for home use are available through Eden Labs (see page 130). These units are quite expensive and will be most useful for the serious hobbyist. However, if you belong to an herb-growing group or garden club with many active members interested in using herbal essences, it may be worth the expense to buy a unit for the members to share.

Coldfinger Herbal Extraction Units are available from

EDEN LABS
Tech Enterprises, Inc.
P.O. Box 4908
Macon, GA 31208
PHONE: 800.293.7648

USES FOR SAGE OIL Essential oil derived from common sage is often used in perfumes, colognes, and aftershaves to provide a subtle, rich undertone that adds depth to light, clear floral and citrus fragrances. Rich in antioxidants, sage oil is also used in shampoos, mouthwash, and toothpastes as well as in deodorants and antiperspirants.

Traditional uses of sage oils and extracts include treatments for digestive problems, respiratory infections, and menstrual disorders. Sage and rosemary gargles were commonly used to soothe sore throats, tongues, and mouths, and sage mouthwash was thought to heal swollen gums. Combined with clove oil, sage gargles were also used to calm the pain of aching teeth.

Breathing in steam can be helpful for those who suffer from sinus, throat, or chest infections. Traditionally, the addition of a few drops of medicinal essential oils such as sage, thyme, and peppermint was thought to assist in healing. Lemon oil not only smells delicious but also helps to deeply open and cleanse facial and neck pores, leaving the skin feeling fresh and smooth.

CAUTION: SAGE OIL IS NOT FOR CONSUMPTION
Although essential oil of sage has many beneficial uses, it is for EXTERNAL USE ONLY. Common sage oil is toxic if ingested. It should NEVER be used in teas or foods of any kind.

OTHER SAGE OILS Several other sages also yield valuable essential oils. Lavender sage oil is used in soaps and as a fixative in potpourri. Clary sage oil, used in church incense, is a fixative in perfumes and adds fragrance to soaps and bath oils.

Sage Steam Facial

Add to a large bowl of steaming hot water:
3 drops sage oil
2 drops peppermint oil
2 drops thyme oil
2 drops lemon oil

Sit over steaming bowl and cover head and bowl with a large towel. Breathe slowly and deeply for 1 minute, matching the length of inhale with equal exhale (to avoid hyperventilating). Remove towel and breath normally for 2 to 3 minutes; then repeat steam treatment for 1 minute.

Sage-Oil Facial Cleanser

3 drops sage oil
2 drops rosemary oil
1 drop lavender oil
1 cup witch hazel extract or astringent

Combine all ingredients and shake well to blend. Store in tightly closed bottle. To use, moisten a cotton ball or pad with a sprinkle of astringent and gently wipe face. In summer, store in the refrigerator and use to cool overheated skin.

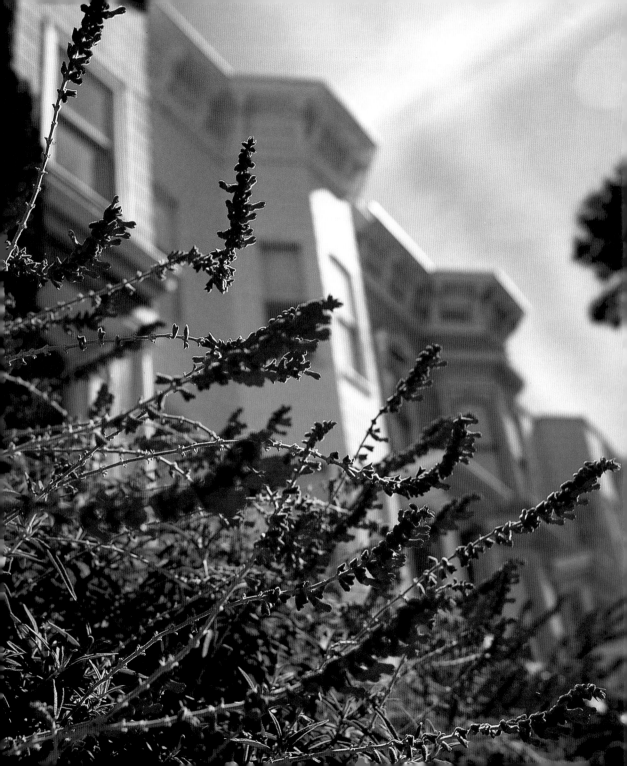

sources *and* resources

Many nurseries carry sages in profusion, but some species and hybrids are hard to track down. The following nurseries carry both edible and ornamental sages.

NURSERY SOURCES FOR SAGES

DIGGING DOG NURSERY
P.O. Box 471
Albion, CA 95410
PHONE: 707.937.1130 (9 AM to 5 PM, Mon.–Sat.)
FAX: 707.937.2480
WEB SITE: www.diggingdog.com
Many sage species
catalog $3; $30 minimum order

GOODWIN CREEK GARDENS
P.O. Box 83
Williams, OR 97544
PHONE: 541.846.7357
FAX: 541.846.7357
WEB SITE: www.goodwincreekgardens.com
Edible and floral species
catalog $1

HIGH COUNTRY GARDENS
2902 Rufina Street
Santa Fe, NM 87505-2929
PHONE: 800.925.9387
FAX: 800.925.0097
WEB SITE: www.highcountrygardens.com
Dryland sages

MILAEGER'S GARDENS
4838 Douglas Avenue
Racine, WI 53402-2498
PHONE: 800.669.9956
FAX: 414.639.1855
WEB SITE: www.milaegers.com
Border sages
catalog $1

NICHOLS GARDEN NURSERY
1190 North Pacific Highway
Albany, OR 97321-4580
PHONE: 541.928.9280
FAX: 800.231.5306
WEB SITE: www.gardennursery.com
Edible and ornamental sages
catalog $2

RENEE'S GARDEN
7389 West Zayante Road
Felton, CA 95018
PHONE: 888.880.7228
FAX: 831.335.7227
WEB SITE: www.reneesgarden.com
Edible and ornamental sages
catalog $1

SISKIYOU RARE PLANT NURSERY
2825 Cummings Road
Medford, OR 97501
PHONE: 541.772.6846
FAX: 541.772.4917
WEB SITE: www.wave.net/upg/srpn
Species and border beauties
catalog s3

THOMPSON & MORGAN INC.
P.O. Box 1308
Jackson, NJ 08527-0308
PHONE: 800.274.7333
FAX: 888.466.4769
Seeds only

WAYSIDE GARDENS
1 Garden Lane
Hodges, SC 29695-0001
PHONE: 800.845.1124
FAX: 800.817.1124
WEB SITE: www.waysidegardens.com
Border beauties

WOODSIDE GARDENS
1191 Egg & I Road
Chimacum, WA 98325
PHONE: 360.732.4754
FAX: 800.453.1152
WEB SITE: www.woodsidegardens.com
Species and border beauties
catalog s2

YUCCA DO NURSERY
P.O. Box 104
Hempstead, TX 77445
PHONE: 409.826.4580
Species and hybrids
catalog s2

books *for* further reading

Sage has been written about so extensively that a complete bibliography would be a book in itself. Here is a selection of recent and classic books that offer useful information about sage and its culinary, herbal, medicinal, and gardenly uses.

Antol, Marie Nadine. *Healing Teas: How to Prepare and Use Teas to Maximize Your Health.* Garden City Park, N.Y.: Avery Publishing Group, 1996.

Armitage, Allan M. *Herbaceous Perennial Plants: A Treatise on Their Identification, Culture and Garden Attributes.* Champaign, Ill.: Stipes Publishing, 1989.

Bacon, Richard M. *The Forgotten Arts: Growing, Gardening & Cooking with Herbs.* Dublin, N.H.: Yankee Publishing, 1972.

Staff of the L. H. Bailey Hortorium, Cornell University. *Hortus Third: A Concise Dictionary of Plants Cultivated in the United States and Canada.* New York: Macmillan Publishing, 1976.

Barton, Barbara. *Gardening by Mail: A Source Book.* New York: Houghton Mifflin, 1997.

Beston, Henry. *Herbs and the Earth: An Evocative Excursion into the Lore & Legend of Our Common Herbs.* Boston: David R. Godine, Publisher, 1995.

Bloomfield, Harold H., M.D. *Healing Anxiety with Herbs.* New York: Harper Collins, 1998.

Brickell, Christopher, and Zuk, Judith D., eds. *The American Horticultural Society A–Z Encyclopedia of Garden Plants.* New York: DK Publishing, 1996.

Bullivant, Elizabeth. *Dried Fresh Flowers.* London: Pelham Books, 1989.

Byers, Dorie. *Herbal Remedy Gardens: 38 Plans for Your Health and Well-Being.* Pownal, Vt.: Storey Communications, 1999.

Clarkson, Rosetta E. *Green Enchantment: The Magic and History of Herbs and Garden Making.* New York: Macmillan Publishing, 1940.

———. *Herbs, Their Culture and Uses: The Complete Guide to Planning, Growing and Harvesting Your Own Herb Garden.* New York: Macmillan Publishing, 1942.

———. *Magic Gardens: A Modern Chronicle of Herbs and Savory Seeds.* New York: Macmillan Publishing, 1939.

Clebsch, Betsy. *A Book of Salvias: Sages for Every Garden.* Portland, Oreg.: Timber Press, 1997.

Clevely, Andy, et al. *The Encyclopedia of Herbs and Spices.* New York: Hermes House, 1997.

Cruden, Loren. *Medicine Grove: A Shamanic Herbal.* Rochester, Vt.: Destiny Books, 1997.

Cunningham, Scott. *Magical Herbalism: The Secret Craft of the Wise.* St. Paul, Minn.: Llewellyn Publications, 1982.

Dodt, Colleen K. *The Essential Oils Book: Creating Personal Blends for Mind & Body.* Pownal, Vt.: Storey Communications, 1996.

Duke, James A., Ph.D. *The Green Pharmacy: New Discoveries in Herbal Remedies for Common Diseases and Conditions.* Emmaus, Pa.: Rodale Press, 1997.

Dumont, Henrietta. *The Floral Offering: The Language and Poetry of Flowers.* Philadelphia: H. C. Peck & Theo. Bliss, 1852.

Ellis, Barbara. *Attracting Birds & Butterflies: How to Plan a Backyard Habitat.* New York: Houghton Mifflin, 1997.

Ettinger, John. *Cooking with Herbs.* Rocklin, Calif.: Prima Publishing, 1996.

Gardiner, Anthony. *Medicinal Oils and Essential Oils.* Edison, N.J., Chartwell Books, 1995.

Gerard, John. *The Herbal or General History of Plants.* New York: Dover Publications, 1975.

Gilbertie, Sal. *Kitchen Herbs: The Art of Enjoyment of Growing Herbs and Cooking Them.* New York: Bantam Books, 1988.

Gordon, Lesley. *Green Magic: Flowers, Plants & Herbs in Lore & Legend.* New York: Viking Press, 1977.

Graves, Robert. *The Greek Myths.* Middlesex, England, Penguin Books, 1955.

———. *The White Goddess.* New York: Farrar, Straus & Giroux, 1948.

Harrar, Sarah, and O'Donnell, Sara Altshul. *The Woman's Book of Healing Herbs: Secrets from 90 Top Herbal Healers.* Emmaus, Pa.: Rodale Press, 1999.

Hedley, Christopher, and Shaw, Non. *Herbal Remedies: A Practical Beginner's Guide to Making Effective Remedies in the Kitchen.* New York: Smithmark Publishers, 1996.

Herbal Research Publications. *Naturopathic Handbook of Herbal Formulas.* Ayer, Mass.: Herbal Research Publications, 1955.

Kowalchik, Claire, and Hylton, William H. *Rodale's Illustrated Encyclopedia of Herbs.* Emmaus, Pa.: Rodale Press, 1998.

Lancaster, Roy. *Travels in China: A Plantsman's Paradise.* Woodbridge, Suffolk, England: Antique Collectors' Club, 1989.

Lawless, Julia. *The Illustrated Encyclopedia of Essential Oils: The Complete Guide to the Use of Oils in Aromatherapy and Herbalism.* New York: Barnes & Noble, 1995.

Lima, Patrick. *The Harrowsmith Illustrated Book of Herbs.* Camden East, Ontario, Canada: Camden House Publishing, 1986.

Mackin, Jeanne. *The Cornell Book of Herbs and Edible Flowers.* Ithaca, N.Y.: Cornell Cooperative Extension, 1993.

Marcin, Marietta Marshall. *The Herbal Tea Garden: Planning, Planting, Harvesting & Brewing.* Pownall, Vt.: Storey Communications, 1983.

Mayell, Mark. *Off-The-Shelf Natural Health: How to Use Herbs and Nutrients to Stay Well.* New York: Bantam Books, 1995.

McIntyre, Anne. *The Good Health Garden: Growing and Using Healing Herbs.* Pleasantville, N.Y.: Reader's Digest Assn., 1998.

——. *The Medicinal Garden: How to Grow and Use Your Own Medicinal Herbs.* New York: Henry Holt & Co., 1997.

Miller, Amy Bess. *Shaker Medicinal Herbs: A Compendium of History, Lore, and Uses.* Pownal, Vt.: Storey Communications, 1998.

Miller, George O. *Landscaping with Native Plants of Texas and the Southwest.* Stillwater, Minn.: Voyageur Press, 1991.

Murray, Michael T., M.D. *The Healing Power of Herbs: The Enlightened Person's Guide to the Wonders of Medicinal Plants.* Rocklin, Calif.: Prima Publishing, 1992.

Norman, Jill. *The Classic Herb Cookbook.* New York: DK Publishing, 1997.

Peterson, Carol R. *More Herbs You Can Master: Twelve Wondrous Plants for: Extra Nutrition, Improved Health, Natural Beauty.* Snoqualmie, Wash.: Mountain Garden Publishing, 1999.

Phillips, Roger, and Foy, Nicky. *The Random House Book of Herbs.* New York: Random House, 1990.

Potterton, David. *Culpepper's Color Herbal.* New York: Sterling Publishing, 1983.

Rawlings, Romy. *Healing Gardens.* Minocqua, Wis.: Willow Creek Press, 1998.

Reader's Digest. *Magic and Medicine of Plants.* Pleasantville, N.Y.: Reader's Digest Assn., 1986.

Schauenberg, Paul, and Paris, Ferdinand. *Guide to Medicinal Plants.* New Canaan, Conn.: Keats Publishing, 1990.

Schultes, Richard Evan, and Hofmann, Albert. *Plants of the Gods: Their Sacred, Healing and Hallucinogenic Powers.* Rochester, Vt.: Healing Arts Press, 1992.

Scully, Virginia. *A Treasury of American Indian Herbs: Their Lore and Their Use for Food, Drugs and Medicine.* New York: Crown Publishers, 1970.

Sedenko, Jerry. *The Butterfly Garden: Creating Beautiful Gardens to Attract Butterflies.* New York: Running Heads, 1991.

Stuart, Malcolm. *The Encyclopedia of Herbs and Herbalism.* London: Orbis Publishing, 1979.

Sturdivant, Lee, and Blakley, Tim. *The Bootstrap Guide to Medicinal Herbs in the Garden, Field & Marketplace.* Friday Harbor, Wash.: San Juan Naturals, 1999.

Sutton, John. *The Gardener's Guide to Growing Salvias.* Portland, Oreg.: Timber Press, 1999.

Valnet, Jean, M.D. *The Practice of Aromatherapy: A Classic Compendium of Plant Medicines & Their Healing Properties.* Rochester, Vt.: Healing Arts Press, 1980.

Weed, Susan S. *Wise Woman Herbal: Healing Wise.* Woodstock, N.Y.: Ash Tree Publishing, 1989.

Weil, Andrew, M.D. *Spontaneous Healing: How to Discover and Enhance Your Body's Natural Ability to Maintain and Heal Itself.* New York: Alfred A. Knopf, 1995.

This map loosely defines the range of average annual minimum temperatures for each zone in degrees ꜰ (note: zones ɪ, ꬶ, and ɪɪ are outside the continental United States). Contact your local garden center for more specific information about your particular climate.

ᴢᴏɴᴇ		
	1	*below* -50°
	2	-50° *to* -40°
	3	-40° *to* -30°
	4	-30° *to* -20°
	5	-20° *to* -10°

ᴢᴏɴᴇ		
	6	-10° *to* 0°
	7	0° *to* 10°
	8	10° *to* 20°
	9	20° *to* 30°
	10	30° *to* 40°
	11	40° *and above*

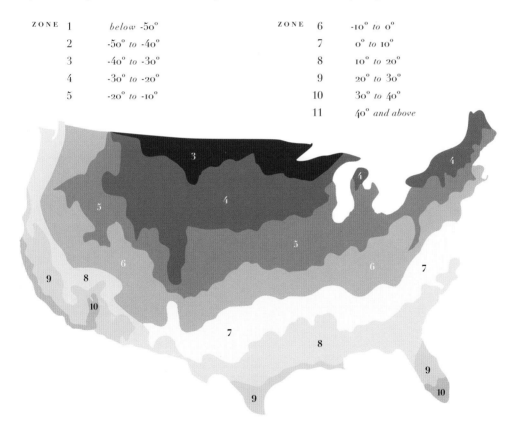

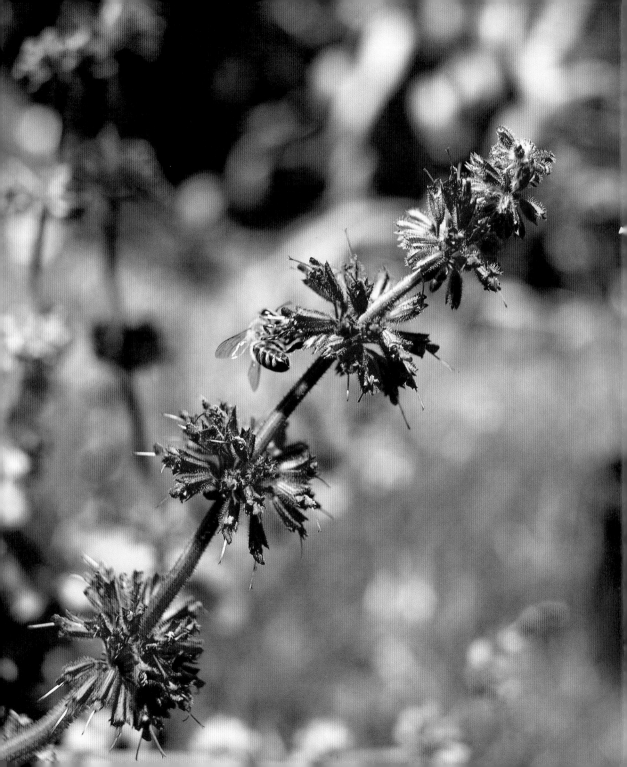

Showy White Bee Common
Wooly Cleveland Gentian Indi
Meadow Spanish Indigo Spire
Blue Purple Rain Mealy Wild
neapple Clary Mexican Roselea
ires Painted Autumn Rosy Me
me Littleleaf Fruit Big Blue Pu
White Bee Common Pineappl
Cleveland Gentian Indigo Spir
panish Indigo Spires Silver Ja
ain Mealy Wild Bog Showy Wh
exican Roseleaf Wooly Clevela
ump Rosy Meadow Spanish